SURVIVING IN STROKE CITY

GERRY ANDERSON
SURVIVING IN STROKE CITY

HUTCHINSON
London

First published in the United Kingdom in 1999
by Hutchinson

Random House (UK) Limited
20 Vauxhall Bridge Road, London SW1V 2SA

Random House Australia (Pty) Limited
20 Alfred Street, Milsons Point, Sydney,
New South Wales 2061, Australia

Random House New Zealand Limited
18 Poland Road, Glenfield,
Auckland 10, New Zealand

Random House South Africa (Pty) Ltd
Endulini, 5A Jubilee Road, Parktown 2193, South Africa

Random House UK Limited Reg. No. 954009

A CIP record for this book is available
from the British Library

Papers used by Random House UK Limited
are natural, recyclable products made from wood grown in
sustainable forests. The manufacturing processes conform to
the environmental regulations of the country of origin.

ISBN 0 09 180064-1

Typeset in Garamond by
MATS, Southend-on-Sea, Essex

Printed and bound in Great Britain by
Clays Ltd, St. Ives plc

To all my family

CONTENTS

Introduction: Hobos and Hubris   1

Death Threats and Other Trivia   10

Dark Corners and Dangling Conversations   22

Anoraks and Anachronisms   37

Drunken Dwarves and Private Thoughts   47

Ego and the Tube   59

Accordions and Chicken Wire   69

Brothers and Others   83

Facts About Fairies   97

Sex and Drugs and On The Dole   110

Dublin Days: a Postscript   157

A 'Celebrity' at the Crossroads   167

White Mice and Maple Syrup   174

'Anderson Country'   191

The Argentinian Returns   206

ANDERSON'S LAW

Sustaining a successful career in showbusiness depends on one's ability to master the art of looking surprised and shocked on being told something that one has already known for some time.

INTRODUCTION:
HOBOS AND HUBRIS

IT WAS THE eyes that got to me.

The shrivelled man sprawled on the pavement was obviously homeless, but his eyes were somewhere else. Somewhere better.

Slowly extending a soiled hand, he muttered something that I didn't quite catch.

Another time I would have strode by, displaying that cold, tight half-smile/half-grimace I had learnt in England for use on occasions such as these. But this time I lingered, and fumbled for small change in my trouser pocket.

Apart from the sparkling eyes he didn't look too good. Wrapped loosely in his Regulation Homeless Man Sleeping Bag that looked as if it had been torn apart by wild animals, he also wore what appeared to be a Mongolian peasant hat complete with ragged peak and moth-eaten earflaps fastened neatly under the chin.

From the debris at the bottom of his sleeping bag protruded two old-fashioned baseball boots that looked as if they had recently exploded, exposing sizeable areas of naked, dirt-encrusted feet.

The other, non-begging hand held the soggy remains of a well-masticated Big Mac. A crumpled packet of Lambert & Butler cigarettes lay by his side in close proximity to a can of Diet Coke.

He was not alone.

A large dog of mixed parentage, with a great lolling tongue and mangy bristling coat that seemed glued unevenly to its stinking hide, glared at me with one good pink eye. The other appeared sightless and resembled a white grape.

The beast was tethered loosely to a convenient drainpipe by means of a loop of the type of intermittently unravelling string that you can't buy any more, string the likes of which I hadn't seen since I was a child.

Anyway, this man, probably in his late thirties, lying in his own filth near the doorway of a swanky jeweller's in Regent Street within dwarf-hurling distance of BBC Broadcasting House in Portland Place, this man curled up against the cruel lash of a late-February north wind, this obvious example of London pondlife, this man whose presence caused passers-by to shudder with a could-that-ever-happen-to-me frisson . . . this wrecked husk of a human being seemed to possess what most of those who bustled by clearly did not have.

Apparent peace of mind.

It was in his eyes. I could see real contentment there.

Nor did this expression of inner well-being seem chemically induced. As an ex-rock musician with some experience in these matters, I could tell that he was dope-free. The facility for spotting stoned people came back to me as that of riding a bicycle. I had once been that soldier, after all.

He beckoned. I approached, clutching an offering of a pound coin.

He chose to speak. His voice had a gentle rasp. 'The wankers are winning worldwide.'

I paused, unsure.

'Fuckin' right,' I replied eventually with some conviction, simultaneously pressing the coin into his hand.

The dog growled and slowly raised its ragged arse two inches off the ground. Poised so, the beast remained perfectly still.

Conversation dried. The homeless one struggled unsteadily to his feet and, without another word, shuffled towards a nearby off-licence, dragging his left foot.

He seemed to leave a trace in his wake . . . like a snail.

I almost envied his uncomplicated life, but most of all I coveted his anonymity.

I was, after all, the Most Hated Man in Britain. I wanted to talk to him about my situation. He'd been through the mill. Maybe he would understand. No one liked him much either would have been my guess. But I didn't hang around for him to come back with his bottle and continued on my way towards the grey stone façade of the BBC clutching the mandatory Corporation briefcase which contained all I needed to survive the day: a dog-eared Filofax, a copy of *Viz* magazine, a packet of anti-smoking patches, twenty Benson & Hedges, a cheese sandwich and a small bottle of red pills, two of which taken every morning made me piss alarmingly every twenty minutes. These had been prescribed by a surly GP with bulging eyes who told me that my occasional dizzy spells would disappear if the fluid level in my inner ear was reduced by means of voluntary dehydration. He didn't mention the side effects, which included a continual powerful lust for strong beer and my facial skin developing the properties of ancient Egyptian papyrus.

It's not easy to become the Most Hated Man in Britain but I had achieved the position swiftly and with remarkable ease. I suppose you could say I was there before I knew it. Having just spent an awkward breakfast reading wounding things about myself in the 'Media' section of the *Guardian*, I was a desperate case.

I wasn't always the Most Hated Man in Britain. Up until recently I was unhated and relatively happy.

Now I was envying hobos.

As a matter of fact, I could safely say that before 21 February 1994, I was reasonably content.

Hitherto I was regarded as a fairly successful TV and radio 'personality' in Northern Ireland and took some pride in the notion that I had, to the best of my knowledge, lost neither my soul nor my dignity in the process.

On radio I was, I suppose, what you might term an anti-

3

broadcaster and didn't particularly go out of my way to be nice to people I didn't like.

It seemed to work, in a way.

I wasn't a shock-jock by any means, but tried in a modest way not to be a Showbiz Wanker.

I took pleasure in the results of a regional poll that sought to discover: (a) who the Northern Ireland public regarded as their favourite broadcaster; and (b) which broadcaster they would most like to see removed from the airwaves.

I was strangely moved and proud to come out top in both categories.

I had a little more trouble on television.

As the 'host' of a weekly Northern Ireland Friday-night chat-show, I found it marginally more difficult to retain a degree of integrity. It's extremely hard not to be a Showbiz Wanker on television because the nature of the medium seems to demand it. I had particular trouble looking interested when talking to people I wasn't interested in, and found it hard to affect hearty laughter when required to do so by a producer who would often scream obscenities deep into my brain via my personal ear-piece. I was particularly uncomfortable with comedians who sat beside me and told jokes in dialect.

I was also often required to look grave when being told grave things by grave people.

I found it hard to care, and appearing not to care is the one unforgivable televisual sin. I came to the conclusion that success in what used to be called light-entertainment television requires supreme self-confidence, complete arrogance, a devious mind and a minimum of intelligence.

Nonetheless, I'm ashamed to admit that I was fairly successful.

I suppose I've always hated showbusiness but, one way or another, I have been in it all my life.

In the seventies I'd been a rock musician in the United States and that was showbusiness too, but somehow it didn't feel like it. There were too many fringe benefits and wonderful opportunities to behave like an animal.

But now I had gone nationwide with Radio 4 in a bid for

glory, and it was all going horribly wrong.

I should have known better. I had tried before.

Before 1990 I had never taken broadcasting seriously, regarding it as a form of remunerative self-therapy, something to do until something else turned up.

I had fallen into radio, as most people do, by accident. Worn out by rock 'n' roll excess in America, I decided to drop out and get myself an education. After four empty years at the New University of Ulster, I emerged clutching a B.Sc.(Hons) in Sociology and Social Anthropology which equipped me for no profession whatsoever.

Undaunted, I eventually talked my way into a job as editor of a small local cross-community magazine in Londonderry called *Community Mirror*. Supremely ignorant concerning all aspects of the newspaper and magazine business, I spent the first day trying to find out how the practical end operated.

The phone rang after I'd been there about twenty minutes.

It was for me.

Someone from the local radio station. 'Hello, BBC Radio Foyle here. Will you do an interview on our afternoon show?' asked the reasonable female voice.

'About what?' I asked.

'Aren't you the new editor?'

'Yes.'

'About that then!' she explained.

'I don't know anything about this magazine,' I confessed.

'So how come you got the job?'

'It wasn't easy.'

'You must know something about it.'

'I don't.'

'Well, do it anyway. It's just a filler.'

'OK then, but don't ask me any questions.'

'I'll have to ask you . . . something!'

'OK, but don't ask me any hard questions . . . like about editorial policy, circulation, reach, advertising revenue, political stance, community issues or any of that stuff. I haven't even read this magazine yet.'

'OK,' she agreed.

I duly appeared at the local radio station, spoke 'live' on air and was, of course, asked all the questions I had asked not to be asked. I filled twenty minutes with glib, shameless lies and when it was over I was approached by the producer, to whom I immediately apologised for the bundle of crap I had just invented.

'You mean you made it all up?'

'Yes, I'm sorry. I asked not to be asked that stuff.'

She whistled slowly, grabbed my arm and took me aside.

'You could be good at this,' she whispered.

So, I became a broadcaster.

I had what it took. I could lie convincingly without apparent effort, fluently and live.

It was easy. I was a late starter for this business. She told me so.

I was forty years old.

No matter.

My career snowballed rapidly after that, and in 1990 I found myself amongst the great and the good at an awards lunch in the Grosvenor House Hotel in London, striding proudly between groaning tables littered with the occasional royal and an unruly horde of dinner-suited well-known radio personalities, on my way to a glittering podium to accept a Sony Gold Award from a smooth-tongued, snowy-headed Michael Aspel, who looked older than I thought he should and didn't know who I was.

I addressed the gathered celebs with humility and left to sustained applause. I was perceived as a refugee from a war zone and had a strong feeling that I was Dr Johnson's fiddling dog, which, in a way, I suppose I was.

I felt important until, clutching my radio Oscar, I was thrown against an elegant flock-papered wall by the Duchess of Kent's bodyguards. I watched her trundle imperiously by.

It was my first brush with royalty but, strangely, not the first time I had been manhandled by representatives of the Crown.

6

As a direct result of being voted Sony Regional Presenter of the Year I was offered a series of Saturday-afternoon shows on Radio 2. I accepted this signal honour and went about the task in a workmanlike manner. The only concession I felt I should make to broadcasting to a predominantly English audience was to speak marginally more slowly on air and say nothing that might alarm household pets or interfere with gardening.

I was to broadcast from the BBC studios in Manchester on Saturday afternoons between the hours of 3.30 and 5.00.

My brief was simple. Play a few records and talk.

My producer was a lachrymose but pleasant man who looked uneasy when I told him that I wouldn't be needing a script of any kind.

When he asked me what I was going to talk about I told him that I didn't know but would think of something when the time came. That was the way I operated, I said.

He accepted that and bade me proceed. He was a solid, decent, intelligent individual from the West Country, and I was greatly encouraged by the fact that he disliked the BBC intensely. It was good to be dealing with someone with a rebellious streak. It's often difficult to communicate with Company Men, whichever company they serve.

In conversation with others, he invariably referred to me as 'The Turn'.

As 'The Turn', I punched in half a dozen shows toning down my act, and only occasionally lapsing into the unacceptable. On the whole, I enjoyed the experience, apart from a minor brush with another member of staff, an in-house producer who subsequently went on to 'greater' things as a frontline presenter on Radio 1.

At that time he seemed a little less than civilised and informed me, during after-show communal drinks, that I was nothing but a fucking Paddy. A man obviously destined to triumph on the rat-wheel.

Apart from this slight unpleasantness, everything was fine and the audience feedback goodish to the extent that another producer with higher connections felt I was ready for greater things. He suggested that it might not be a bad idea to have a crack at the Radio 2 flagship Breakfast Show, at that time under the stewardship of the garrulous Derek Jameson. The plan was to slip me in for two or three weeks whilst Derek was on holiday and see how things went.

I assumed that words were exchanged at the highest level, and as a consequence I was summoned to London for an audience with the Controller of Radio 2.

At the appointed date I made my way through the large wooden doors of Broadcasting House and was met by a flunky who led me up lifts and down long corridors into the imposing lair of the Controller, who greeted me stiffly.

The Controller of Radio 2 was a tidy, outwardly friendly woman with a hawkish mien. She was in her late forties and obviously took no prisoners.

I sat politely facing her across a highly polished desk.

'I've been listening to your programmes,' she began.

'Yes?' I replied.

'Not bad.'

'Thank you.'

'Do you listen to radio much?'

'Not if I can help it,' I replied, truthfully, but probably unwisely.

She settled her elbows on her desk-top and studied me intently. 'These are challenging times. Radio 2 has to keep up with what is happening.'

'Well, what *is* happening?'

'More music stations, less speech. We have to move with the times and give the public what it wants.'

'And what does the public want?' I asked in all innocence.

'In a manner of speaking, music without speakers. Music that our listeners are comfortable with. Less DJ prattle.'

'Well, somebody has to say something.'

'Not beyond telling the listeners what they're listening to.'

The station was struggling at the time and had done so since the departure of the Great Wogan to the flesh-pots of television.

'You mean, "Good morning, ladies and gentlemen, what a beautiful day this is. Reminds me of '67, the Summer of Love, and what better to kick off with than 'Let's Go to San Francisco'?" and then after that: " '67! What a year that was! Here's the Hollies." Is that the road you intend to go down?'

'More or less,' she replied quietly, I think a tad embarrassed.

'I think you're making a mistake. You're taking the Roy Orbison Trail. It's the road to nowhere.'

'It's working for the others,' she said.

(But we're not the others. We're the fucking BBC, for Chrissakes. You say you want music without speakers. You just don't have the speakers that people want to listen to. You need fewer tweedy wankers and hollow men. Fewer smug, fat-cat golfers masquerading as deejays. You need someone to give the listeners the unexpected, somebody half-human, somebody who has lived in the real world, someone with an attitude. Then they'll listen!)

At least, that's what I said in my own mind.

What I really said was, 'Isn't there a possibility you could be mistaken?'

'No,' she replied.

'Well, then. If that's the way you intend to go, I don't see much room for the likes of me. I'm a speaker.'

'Quite,' she murmured.

She rose and made her way towards the door. 'It's been lovely meeting you,' she said gushingly, throwing me a cold smile and extending the limp hand of farewell.

I had learnt a valuable lesson.

Never be in the right place at the wrong time.

People don't like you for it.

DEATH THREATS AND
OTHER TRIVIA

I ONCE KNEW an old man from a long since razed area of
Belfast who eked out a living shaving dead pigs' cheeks with
an old-fashioned cut-throat razor. At any one sitting he rarely
shaved two cheeks belonging to the same pig and if by chance
he ever did minister to a matching set of porcine jowls,
chances were he would have been unaware of it.

This was because, not so long ago, the people of Northern
Ireland found it convenient to purchase half a pig's head cut
longways. This was a handy size for the average pot, made
exceptional stock and had the advantage of having only the
one eye stare out at the cook when he or she lifted the lid to
monitor the boiling process. Two steaming, staring eyes can
be scary.

Sheep's heads, on the other hand, were prepared exclusively
for consumption by greyhounds, but remained unshaven due
to problematical logistics.

But that's another story.

The pig-shaver's craft was necessary for reasons that will
appear immediately obvious. There are certain things a living
pig cannot do on its own, and it is generally accepted that the
average porker can be depended on neither to fly nor to shave
on a regular basis.

Consequently when a pig is dispatched it is normally found
to be sporting a fairly impressive five o'clock shadow, which
is good news for the pig-shaver kept busy at the strop for the

benefit of the general public, who don't usually fancy stubbled pork for lunch.

All in the past, of course, in times more austere. Another cottage industry bites the dust.

But who's to shave a pig's cheek these days? It seems an indecent question to ask the average supermarket check-out girl, who'll look blankly through you with long-dead eyes.

The art of comfortable communication is foundering.

People don't talk to each other like they used to, but they do listen to the radio more than they did. I talk on BBC Radio Ulster every morning, and some of the people out there listen and occasionally talk back to me.

I hear about a man from Andersonstown in Belfast who specialised in shortening puppies' tails on a piece-work basis. He was untrained in veterinary science but discovered he had a knack for it. He was very good . . . a natural. Everybody said so and no dog was heard to as much as whimper when the blade unerringly fell. Just a quick chop and it was done. He always got it exactly right.

His name was Jack.

I also do requests. I get letters sent from prisons written by people who have planted bombs that have blown up other people. They want me to say hello to their loved ones and play something by Jim Reeves or Daniel O'Donnell. I don't usually oblige, for the simple reason that I am reasonably sure that the relatives of those they have blown up will be listening too. Doesn't do to offend.

It's a small country and many people don't like each other.

Most daily radio shows trudge a well-worn road of competitions, quizzes, weather and travel updates, gardening hints, money-management tips, celebrity gossip, honk your horn if having an enema, put a bet on this horse today, horoscopes for the brain-dead, two tracks from a classic album, name the mystery object making this sound !!!!, did-you-know-that-Adolf-Hitler-was-born-on-this-day-one-hundred-years-ago? kind of shit and other items designed to drive sensible people insane. Music calculated not to startle the innocent is selected beforehand and a running order is established with the aforementioned items of perceived interest inserted at timely intervals.

I do none of these things and am proud to say that my programme has no planned content.

It goes without saying that an untrammelled radio tongue is a dangerous thing to employ within the confines of Northern Ireland, populated as it is by too many gun-totin' crazy people who believe God is on their side.

These people are quick to take offence.

It is important at all times to be aware of who might be listening and with what kind of ears, because, in our troubled statelet, diverse ears hear different things. Some extremely finely tuned ears hear things that haven't been said at all. An example is called for . . .

Not so long ago in the course of my daily duties I had occasion to play a fairly toe-curling version of a song called 'Deck of Cards', performed by a singer with the surprising name of Wink Martindale. You know the song, of course . . . Second World War soldier in North African campaign is apprehended in church by superior officer for producing sinful playing cards during service . . . threatened by punishment worse than death (your own mother won't know you, etc.) unless he can explain himself . . . humble grunt explains patiently that the deck of cards remain his only means of religious solace during battle and bouts of grindingly difficult forced marches through shimmering sand dunes and worse . . . the numbered and the face cards keep him in touch with treasured Biblical occurrences, e.g. the nine reminds him of the ten lepers cured by Jesus (only one thanked Him and therefore didn't count as an ingrate) . . . the eight reminds him of the eight people spared in the suburbs of Sodom and Gomorrah (make that nine if Lot's wife had looked straight ahead) . . . penny finally drops and lowly faithful cannon fodder is forgiven by soft-hearted superior officer and probably given twenty-four hours' R&R in Cairo . . . you know, the usual bollocks.

Anyway, the narrator ends with the line, 'I know, for I was that soldier.' All in all, just your average innocent dollop of sentimental gunge. Innocent enough in itself.

When the record was over, I said, 'See me? See soldiers? I hate them.'

This is quite a common mode of speech in Northern Ireland. Grammatically suspect though it may be, its origins can be found in the Ulster-Scots blood that infects many of our citizens. If, for example, I don't care for, say, sugar, I would say, 'See me? See sugar? I hate it.' It's essentially BillyConnollyspeak.

By making the comment I suppose I was merely expressing a general distaste for any form of warmongering. As far as I was concerned, it was a perfectly innocent peacenik remark. I couldn't have been more wrong. A great number of listeners immediately accused me of castigating the British Army in Northern Ireland. I had finally come out ... laid myself bare and exposed my true feelings. I had emerged from the closet as a man who hated the British Army and was there-fore, by definition, a Nationalist slimeball. A crypto-Fascist card-carrying-IRA, power-hungry, child-molesting slogan-screaming menace to society. I had many calls to prove it. This lasted for weeks. I received death threats by post, invariably misspelt, and scrawled in that black, black ink that nobody uses any more.

These threats came from Protestant/Loyalist sources, presumably because they had reason to like the Army at the time. Allegiances can shift daily. Sometimes Nationalists/ Catholics like the Army too, but usually everybody hates Her Majesty's Forces at the same time ... for different reasons. Synchronised hate.

As a general rule, Nationalists/Catholics hate the Army because they feel badgered and persecuted unnecessarily by soldiers from another country who 'shouldn't be in Ireland at all', and Protestants/Loyalists hate the Army because they feel Nationalists/Catholics aren't being badgered and persecuted half enough.

It's a wonderful country.

Things got worse.

I was, at the time, involved with a fairly controversial Saturday-night television show that unwisely operated on the premise that a little satirical fun poked at local politicians could do nothing but good.

The programme went out live late on Saturday night, and during afternoon rehearsals we were subjected to a bomb scare. This was a fairly common occurrence at the time, so we all dutifully and routinely filed out of the building until the all-clear was given . . . standard procedure.

As we eventually trickled back, I was taken aside and brought upstairs to the production office, where I was told by the producer that he had received a call from the RUC.

'They say they've received a death threat,' he said, smiling thinly.

'Anybody we know?' I replied breezily.

'You.'

There was a silence.

'They told the police you're next. They say they're going to shoot you,' he revealed.

'Why?'

'They didn't say.'

'Who are "they"?'

'Loyalists, apparently.'

Sweat formed above my upper lip. It was important to remain calm. I searched for words.

'Any kind of time scale here?' I asked weakly.

'They didn't say.'

'Tonight?'

'They didn't say. Police reckon maybe.'

'Did they use a password?'

'Yeah.'

'Genuine?'

'Kosher.'

'What did the police say I should do?'

'They say it's up to you. They'll send somebody in plain

clothes to keep an eye on you tonight but you won't know who it is.'

'What would you do if you were in my position?' I asked.

'I don't know. I've never been in that situation. If I were you I'd do the show, though. If you don't, the story will get out and you'll attract attention.'

He fiddled with his pen and avoided my desperate gaze.

Anger welled within my frightened frame.

I cracked somewhat.

'And what do you call this? I call this attracting attention! They're going to SHOOT me, for fuck's sake! That's what I call attracting fucking attention!'

I was beginning to disintegrate.

He tried to soothe me.

'The police will frisk everybody coming in. You'll be all right. Just get tonight over with and talk to the police tomorrow. Nothing else you can do.'

Easy for him to say.

It was my arse on the line.

'Suppose there is no tomorrow? Who will I talk to then?'

'They're not going to shoot you dead live on television. Why would they do that?' he rasped unconvincingly.

'Ever heard of PR? Think of the mileage they'd get out of that. It would be shown on every TV station in the world. The only properly lit murder ever!'

I was not convinced, but nevertheless decided the show must go on ... this was showbusiness after all and we were nothing if not professionals.

It is said that there is nothing more stressful than live television, but I'm bound to say that dressing-room nerves are considerably exacerbated by the added expectation of being mown down during transmission by some born-again crazed gunman.

I took solace in a half-bottle of vodka.

It was the only way.

The show was housed in a barn-like set designed as an expansive cabaret club complete with dance floor, well-spaced tables, chairs and a real bar serving real alcohol.

A balcony loomed ominously above, it too replete with tables and chairs ... all in all much space for cameras and audience to move about freely.

The audience usually numbered 150 souls and, of course, it was too late to vet the punters properly. They would be arriving soon with tickets in hand, and God knows it would have been easy enough for a man with evil intentions to get his hands on one.

Arrangements were made whereby the audience were heartily frisked at the door by gorillas and I was assured that a plain-clothes person would shadow my every move, but I was not comforted by the knowledge that members of the audience could roam freely about the set and were usually half-pissed before they got there anyway.

The vodka bottle was empty by transmission time and I didn't appear until the last possible moment. The audience was in place. Let somebody else warm the bastards up.

The opening theme music blared and I darted through a glittering door, assuming my position at the top of a flight of awkward stairs down which I was scheduled to confidently stride. The heat from the studio lights and the vodka hit me simultaneously. I wobbled down on what felt like somebody else's legs. Sweat streamed from every pore and the room danced crazily.

With a glassy smile I hit my mark and found I couldn't focus on the autocue. I was drunk, with nothing to say.

I gabbled some slurred nonsense and an acrobat materialised. It was that kind of show.

My opening link done, I was ushered away by the floor manager and steered towards the bar, where my next link was due to be delivered.

I teetered there with some trepidation. This area contained the bulk of the audience and, in the grip of extreme paranoia, I imagined my assassin was near.

As I reached the epicentre of the mob I noticed with horror that a man with one hand lodged in his inside jacket pocket was edging towards me. He had trouble weaving through the crowd but was definitely heading my way.

I found myself hemmed in by the multitude closing in behind, trying to get their ugly faces on camera.

My head spun as I caught his eye.

His face was a mask of determination. He was mere yards away.

He was almost on top of me.

I reeled back as far as I could. He withdrew his hand slowly from his inside pocket.

I caught a glimpse of something dark, and a silent scream formed in my throat.

Suddenly he was on the floor being sat upon by a burly, long-haired man wearing blue jeans and a checked shirt. Women screamed and men craned their necks to see the action. The young man who had rugby-tackled him wrested an object from my would-be assailant's hand.

It was a black, leather-bound autograph book . . .

The poor punter was being sat upon by the authorised thug I now knew to be the man detailed to look after me.

I felt better after that and, as they say in this part of the world, the night passed over peaceful.

At the end of the show I was still alive . . . just.

Weeks of worry and sleepless nights followed and, as is the way of these things, the passage of time dulled my dread to the extent that eventually I no longer feared hourly for my life and only occasionally checked the underside of my car in the morning lest it had a bomb attached . . . the new Highway Code.

Remember, this was only a few years ago, when extreme individuals from both sides of the political divide felt it their duty to shoot babies, blow up hospitals and schools, kill husbands and fathers in their beds or whilst they were watching television with their families.

A fellow had to watch his step.

Sometimes people were murdered by mistake and per-functory, useless apologies were issued to bereaved relatives by representatives of the inadequately informed hitmen.

'Sorry about that, missus, they thought your son was somebody else . . . just one of those things.'

A person had to try and make sense of it.

It wasn't easy.

I was reviled in some quarters for changing the name of the city from which I broadcast. The name of the city is Londonderry. Perhaps a little background is necessary.

People have been living in our city for 1,500 years . . . not the same people, of course; it just sometimes feels that way.

Originally a monastic settlement peopled by darting ascetic monks, by the tenth century the place had a real name . . . Doire Colmcille – 'Doire' being Gaelic for 'oak grove' and 'Colmcille' the name of the peripatetic founding saint of the parish.

Over the following few centuries 'Doire Colmcille' became simplified and anglicised to plain 'Derry'.

In the early seventeenth century the area was developed by a number of London companies and tradesmen's guilds, resulting in the 1613 Charter of Incorporation that officially changed the name of the city to Londonderry in honour of these running dogs of capitalism. The native Catholic Irish were cleared off the land like vermin, and stout Scottish and English folk were 'planted' and given as much land as they could shake a stick at. A sturdy wall was built around the city for the long-term protection of the 'Planters', and the fun began. As one can readily see, this was no blueprint for good community relations in the future. After many years of insurrection, siege and random slaughter, an uneasy co-existence developed, with Protestants referring to the city as Londonderry, and Catholics preferring to use the traditional Derry.

With the inevitable passage of time, distinctions were blurred and soon everybody called the city Derry simply because it was easier to say.

Come the present 'Troubles'.

A new era dawned in the 1980s and a group of people with

a Nationalist bent managed to gain control of the local council and as a gesture of dubious goodwill changed its name to Derry City Council, thereby alienating the entire Protestant population, who thereafter, as a matter of principle, insisted on calling the city by its proper name of Londonderry, even though they had never done so before. The poor old battered Catholics, knowing no better, continued to call the city Derry, as they always had. The very name of the city subsequently became a cudgel with which to beat one's neighbours.

A beast was born.

So it came to pass that a person's religion could almost certainly be ascertained by asking that person to utter the name of the city in which he or she lived.

During recent dark days, when people were randomly killed or seriously interfered with because of their religious affiliation, one can see the importance of hedging one's bets and the desirability of having a sporting chance.

Picture a lonely road in the dead of night. A man is driving wearily home only to observe ahead the sinister outline of shady figures in the middle of the road wielding bobbing flashlights. He stops and winds down his window . . . he has little choice. It could be a legitimate check-point. But maybe not.

A shadowy figure asks him where he is from.

His life may depend on the answer. If the interrogators are looking for a Protestant to work out on, a reply of 'Derry' may be enough to be granted a welcome gruff 'Off you go, then.' If it's bad luck to be a Catholic that night, a 'Derry' could be enough to seal a man's fate.

To circumnavigate this formidable obstacle, the BBC mandarins decreed that presenters on radio and television, faced with the onerous task of having to articulate the name of the city, should at first utterance use 'Londonderry' and thereafter, in the same broadcasting segment, the abbreviation 'Derry'.

I, numbed by the complexity of this, took to naming the

city Derry Stroke Londonderry until ultimately settling for the more natural, user-friendly 'Stroke City'.

To my surprise, this new usage rapidly caught on and became a handy get-out for those challenged by thuggish strangers to name their native city. And so I managed to make enemies of all those who thought that the choice of the pointed use of 'Derry' or 'Londonderry' as a matter of principle at all times was of great importance.

For supplying sensible people with an alternative I was heartily disliked by a sizeable and dangerous proportion of Stroke City and beyond.

But I wasn't on the radio to be liked by everybody. I knew that now.

So what if every once in a while I innocently upset the Bible-thumpers?

So what if I happened to speculate that if Jesus Christ really did love the little children he would have given them some decent weather to play in rather than condemn them to sit indoors in foul weather forced to watch *Neighbours* and *Home and Away*? So what if I am corrected on air by some zealot who maintains that the evidence proving Jesus really does love the little children is contained in the Bible, namely in: Matthew, Chapter 18 Verse 6, also in Chapter 19 Verses 13–14; and Mark, Chapter 10 Verses 13–16?

I checked them myself. No mention whatsoever in there of any Australian soap.

So what if a scoutmaster from Bangor comes to the conclusion that I'm filthy scum and tells me so?

So what if I suggest that the Blessed Virgin may not be a great judge of character on the flimsy evidence that one of the blessed young boys to whom she divinely appeared at the Yugoslavian Holy Place of Medjugorge is now fleecing the tourists by means of various sophisticated scams?

This is a land of incoming flak and Biblical fundamentalism. A land inhabited by people who look alike but who are separated by medieval shibboleths, the origins of which they are but dimly aware, prodded on by slimy leaders who know that the slightest tug on the tail of distant folk memory will produce the desired unruly results.

A green land dotted by cities and towns of grey.

DARK CORNERS AND DANGLING
CONVERSATIONS

PHILIP LARKIN ONCE wrote that sex wasn't invented in Ireland until 1963. I feel the same way about colour. Early days in Stroke City always appeared grey to me.

The sky was grey, buildings were grey, and so were dogs, cats, my uncle's overcoat and trilby hat, women's nylons, pig's feet, people's faces, wood, socks and rugs. For some reason most cars were black, but some were grey. Everything else was grey too . . . to me.

Stroke City was a thriving port and, yes, the sea was battleship grey and so were . . . ah . . . the battleships and destroyers that lined the wharves and disgorged the scum of the waves to drink and carouse in my city of grey.

The only slash of colour I remember was the pigmentation of Gretta Torren's profane parrot domiciled at the top of our street . . . an exotic creature that spent most of its time securely indoors encased in its guano-encrusted cage.

At certain times of the year the parrot was trundled outdoors and its cage hung carefully head-high on the wall beside Gretta's front door. The parrot's outdoor presence usually coincided with the disembarkation of Scottish visitors from the good ship *Laird's Loch* which docked at the bottom of our street after an overnight passage from Glasgow.

These Scottish visitors invariably streamed past Gretta's door on their way to catch a bus to Donegal and would often remark on the surface beauty of the parrot.

But woe to the native Scot who would prod an inquisitorial naked finger within beak range.

At the merest hint of 'Prrrretty Pooolly, Prrrretty Pooooolly,' the parrot would reply with a guttural though clearly enunciated instruction to 'Fuck off!'

On the assumption that the parrot had been specially trained to abuse Scottish people, the bird was eventually impounded by the police.

Like the parrot, I didn't much care for Scottish people either. Strange. As a rule, I don't often agree with parrots.

Stroke City was a strange, silent town, sulking about its history. The spires of two great cathedrals towered disapprovingly over a disaffected, beaten population.

Decades of resentment spilt on to the streets in the late sixties and early seventies, when youths and grown men would spend many a fun-filled hour hurling rocks at British soldiers. The young activists would ape their elders, throwing smaller rocks at the shorter soldiers, each direct hit drawing an approving whoop from the ever-present band of non-participating spectators.

Then it all went wrong when the big boys came out to play. People got killed, and soon, after dark, the streets were empty except for the scurrying of the surly, rat-like young. Reasonable people stopped assembling riotously as a form of recreation and returned to their firesides, to howl fruitlessly at the moon in the privacy of their own homes. The nightmare began.

Even the night-walkers disappeared. Stroke City had always been rich in the quality and variety of its nocturnal wanderers, haunted men who, for no apparent good reason, paced the streets endlessly in the small hours in search of fellow travellers.

Most of these were tortured, intelligent but poorly educated souls who had long ago been left behind by a streamlined, discriminatory education system.

Northern Ireland, in the bad old days when it governed

itself, had a habit of creating far too many of these men ...
men who had never been afforded an opportunity to fulfil
their potential. Most didn't realise they'd been thrown on to
the garbage heap until it was too late, and some of them took
it badly.

In a run-down area near the centre of town stood a ram-
shackle shop of sorts that stayed open until five o'clock in the
morning. It was part pawn shop, part second-hand clothes-
sorting area, but, most importantly, a café that sold no food.
One could, however, purchase a fetid cup of tea served in a
dangerously grimy cup with semi-solid sediment oozing from
its base.

The place was owned and operated by Peggy, who made
little or no money for her pains but seemed to receive her
reward in other ways. She held court behind a shop counter
piled feet-high with assorted dingy crockery, pots, pans,
dusty books, extinct magazines, musty items of clothing,
second-hand rat-traps, rubber hot-water bottles, worn shoes,
damaged lampshades, detachable pick-ups for electric guitars,
the occasional battered fiddle, old Thermos flasks and a large,
surprisingly agile, ginger tomcat called Pinky.

Elsewhere there were wardrobes, washboards with glass
fronts, hand-operated mangles, a dented trumpet, half of a
trombone, and a cast-iron object that I swear was a
ploughshare.

Everything was for sale, though I never once witnessed
anything being sold.

Amongst this triumph of variety and pointlessness stood
the imperious Peggy.

Her own grubby clothes habitually smelt of stale piss, and
she loved to talk.

Not just any old talk.

Not just any old gossip.

She preferred good, stimulating, difficult talk.

She was particularly fond of discussing Darwin's Theory of
Evolution and its effect upon the perceived truths of the
Roman Catholic Church. She also had a soft spot for

Einstein's Theory of Relativity and the subsequent possibility of time travel. Endless hours were spent discussing hypotheses purporting to explain why a stick appears to bend alarmingly when it is immersed in water, or why the sky is blue.

This was what the night-wanderers wanted, and this was where they gathered.

Nobody knew what the fuck they were talking about, but it somehow felt good, almost intellectual.

Peggy's was an escape from the empty darkness of their lives.

I discovered Peggy's at a relatively tender age, whilst I was reeling home drunkenly after fruitlessly groping a girl called Dympna who worked in a shirt factory.

I had walked her back from a dance hall and, grossly over-estimating my personal charisma due to a surfeit of cheap, potent wine, had invested much time talking to her before making an ill-judged lunge at her person. Forcibly repelled, I staggered away at the pointed slamming of her front door.

Fending off a puke, I found myself staring through a dimly illuminated shop front, surprised to see people not only still up, but engaged in animated conversation. I lurched in, mumbling about needing something warm to lean against, and was given leave to stand unsteadily within the confines of the emporium, where I saw and heard enough to want to return sober at a later date.

I subsequently returned frequently to Peggy's talking shop. Nights well spent.

It's all gone now, of course. An anonymous shopping centre now squats on the site.

But the ghosts still linger.

I see Blind Eddie peer inquisitively over the top of the newspaper that he holds two inches in front of his face in a doomed attempt to render the headlines more clear to his almost sightless eyes. He is wearing a long, shapeless, moth-eaten Crombie coat and his hedgehog-grey-flecked hair is on back-to-front.

Thin John leans awkwardly on the counter, toying with his

germ-ridden cup of tea. A felt cap is pulled almost halfway down his face and he is wearing surprising trousers that dangle too far above a pair of steel-capped hobnail boots. He sports a huge white plastic hearing aid on his left ear and wires trail from it to some battery-powered device secreted in the vicinity of the lapel of his soup-stained jacket. A stilted conversation is therefore going on between Peggy, a man who can see very little, and a man who can't hear much at all.

If we include Peggy's severe limp, I am the only person present who is more or less functioning normally.

Peggy speaks in a clipped, fussy tone. 'I was reading a most interesting article in *National Geographic* the other day about cargo cults. Ever heard of them?' Her lips purse in a superior manner.

I am sitting on a pile of mice-gnawed old clothes, idly flicking through a year-old copy of *Exchange & Mart*.

'Pardon?' says Thin John.

'Ever heard of them? Cargo cults?' Peggy repeats.

Blind Eddie squints at the wall and mumbles to himself.

Thin John has heard.

'Ah, yes, cargo cults!' he cries.

'Heard of them?' enquires Peggy again.

'I think I have,' muses Thin John. 'Isn't a cargo cult a form of quasi-religious movement that used to be practised in remote West Indian or African native settlements based on initial contacts with the aeroplane of the white man?'

'Well, sort of,' huffs Peggy.

Thin John becomes animated. 'And when the Europeans landed, weren't the natives more impressed by the stuff the white man hauled out of his plane rather than by his main message of Eternal Salvation?'

'What kind of stuff?' enquires Blind Eddie.

'Y'know ... beads, red flannel, hand mirrors, right up the scale to agricultural implements and maybe whiskey or even jukeboxes, for all I know.'

Blind Eddie looks puzzled and screws up his eyes tightly. 'What period are we talking about here?'

'Late nineteenth century. The Scramble for Africa.'

'Were there planes then?'

Thin John snorts contemptuously. 'Don't nitpick! Anyway, it turned out, didn't it, that the natives weren't all that surprised to receive a visit from strange men who came down from the sky, because that kinda fitted the primitive theology that most of them shared. Basically, like ourselves, they believed that there must be something up there somewhere to explain why everybody is down here looking up! Follow me?'

Blind Eddie harrumphs.

Thin John continues.

'But it wasn't the white men that impressed them, per se . . . It was the cargo that bowled them over, the goodies the white man had brought with him. So, when the white men went away, the natives revised their beliefs and adjusted their rituals so that the material goods became the main object of worship. Just like ourselves, they wanted more stuff, so they prayed for whiskey and washing machines and God knows what else and erected shrines to material goods, cults founded on the worship of Stuff. Forget the Big Fellow. Cut out the middleman. Cargo cults. Get it?'

There is a strained silence. I sense that Thin John has said something out of line but my antennae have not picked it up. Peggy turns away slowly and does something I have never seen her do before. She washes two tea-cups.

Blind Eddie comes to life. 'So what you're saying is that the natives in Africa are just like us because they always want more stuff.'

'In a manner of speaking, I suppose. Yes.'

'Well, we're not the same as them. We're Christians,' Eddie says confidently.

'Christians my arse!' I venture. 'What do you think Christianity is anyway? Just another means of social control, that's what. It's all the same. Protestant Christians, Catholic Christians, Hindus, Buddhists, Jains. No difference.'

'Hold on!' cries John, holding up a stricken hand. 'I didn't mean to suggest that Catholics were the same as Protestants.'

'Of course they are. No difference,' I reply.

There is a sharp intake of breath audible around the rancid room.

'No difference at all!' I continue. 'The purpose of Christianity is to keep poor people in their place by telling them that if they behave themselves they will be rewarded in heaven when they're dead. This allows rich people to gather more stuff without having to worry about poor people taking it away from them. And it works for poor people too, because even if they have little or no stuff, their neighbours won't steal it because their religion tells them that it's wrong to take other people's stuff. Social control, that's all it is.

'If everybody's religious it means you get to keep whatever little stuff you have. It's all about keeping stuff. And it's the same all over the world . . . even in fuckin' Africa!'

Peggy intervenes quietly to say that she doesn't think that is the kind of talk she wants to hear in her shop.

I say it is her fault because she started it by talking about cargo cults.

She says if she had known I was going to talk about Protestants and Catholics she would never have mentioned the subject at all. She doesn't want anybody to get upset.

She asks me to leave.

I leave.

I came back the next night, though, and cargo cults were never mentioned again, although we did make passing reference to the pros and cons of believing in the Transubstantiation of the Holy Eucharist.

What a marvellous country this is. Even the uneducated people know nothing.

Stroke City needed places like Peggy's; places that reflected a country that was standing still in time.

There is, as it happens, still extant a pub we shall call Benny's that operates on the same principles as Peggy's.

It's not hard to find. Self-contained premises stand wearily on a barren street corner amid the remains of buildings long ago bombed and vandalised by local self-appointed 'freedom fighters' who were creating a new and better Ireland by the tried and trusted method of destroying homes inhabited by the unemployed.

It's a real pub in the old style. Stifling air hangs heavy with dust, and walls, ceilings and fittings are forty shades of the same dirty brown.

Benny's is owned and run by two shuffling, elderly bachelor brothers whose world-weary, baggy eyes peer slyly from no-man's land behind the gloomy bartop. Encased in threadbare woollen cardigans, grubby shirts and food-stained ties, they oversee their territory with a degree of detachment, disdain and deliberate movement worthy of some of the older Galapagos tortoises.

The two have been together so long that they have ceased to communicate with each other via the spoken word. We're talking telepathy here.

An imperceptible nod of a head from one brother to the other will result in the opening of a small window for the purpose of letting in a little rancid air. A barely discernible twitch of a pinky or, perhaps, a slightly raised left eyebrow will prompt a brother to disappear through the hanging bead curtain which seductively conceals their private communal living quarters.

He will return after a respectable period of time bearing a toasted bacon sandwich, which will be consumed quietly by the other brother, his eyes lightly scanning the desperate customers. I'm there too, trying to crack the code.

I toy with the notion that they are not really communicating at all and that everything just happens at the same time every day . . . automatically.

I run with this theory for a week or so, until my hypothesis is proved unsound by the instance of an electric fire being turned on at two o'clock in the afternoon round about the time the floor behind the bar is usually swept by one brother or another using the pub witch's broom, but I reckon I'm getting close.

It'll come as no surprise when I tell you that no women are allowed to cross Benny's threshold, no matter what the law of the land decrees. This law is rigorously enforced. But if some foolhardy, ignorant or drunken soul does happen to risk squiring a lady on to the premises, he is treated in much the same way as a child molester would be greeted in Wormwood Scrubs.

I have witnessed transgressions of this nature. The couple enter unaware, like as not laughing happily. Before they get a chance to settle, the brothers exchange looks of alarm. One will then dart under the bar-flap, re-emerge on the customer side and, in the manner of a policeman making an arrest, gently shoo the couple to a spot near the door.

After a brief mumbled exchange, a patronising friendly arm is wrapped around the woman's shoulder and she is calmly steered in the direction of the street. Her escort doesn't usually protest, sensing that he is in the midst of something preternatural of which he should not be critical.

The threat repelled, the brother returns, smiling sheepishly. This is the cue for scattered manly guffaws and some spirited crotch-scratching. Maybe, for emphasis, one or two telling gobs of spit will be propelled noisily to the floor.

The joyful moment fades quickly and silence once again descends like a shroud.

Men drink here to get away from women and don't want to be reminded of them. There is some occasional animated conversation amongst the customers but the prevailing sound is that of poor-quality musak played on one of those long-forgotten eight-track cartridges which elsewhere have become completely extinct.

I once mentioned this background drone to one of the brothers.

'You know, I have a few of those old eight-track cartridges lying at the bottom of an old cardboard box at home,' I said. 'You might like them. Vary the musical diet a bit.'

His eyes flickered with momentary interest and he leaned forward, clutching the rim of the bar with bony pipe-stem arms.

'Really?' he replied in a nasal whine. 'Any words on them?'

'What do you mean?' I asked.

'Words. Are there singers singing words on them?'

I laughed. 'Of course there are words on them. I've got a nice Frank Sinatra, a bit of Nat King Cole and I think Doris Day's in there somewhere too. Just the thing for in here. I'll drop them in if you like.'

'Don't bother,' he said. 'They're of no use to me. I only play music without words. Words distract and sometimes alter the flow of a conversation.'

He cocked his right ear.

'Listen to that,' he whispered.

There was indeed a faint hum of conversation. The general topic, as far as I could make out, was the lack of interest shown by the young in the sport of greyhound racing.

'This is good healthy man's talk,' the brother said. 'If I had Frank Sinatra singing in here, maybe a line from some song he was singing would catch the ear of somebody talking and put him off his flow. Maybe a line about lost love or women or something stupid like that. Something that might depress him by reminding him of a personal episode that he would rather not recall.'

He turned away and absent-mindedly polished a pint glass.

As I scanned a clientele comprised almost exclusively of obvious losers I figured he was probably right.

He wasn't a publican. He was a therapist.

Perched two stools from me was Jack, a morose man in his late seventies. He sat, as he always did, with an unlit pipe clenched in his toothless mouth, taking very occasional tiny sips from the pint of Bass before him, whilst engaged in his permanent occupation. This involved staring straight ahead into the middle distance.

Jack didn't talk much and wanted to be left alone. He was a Second World War veteran and had things on his mind. For reasons best known to himself, he never talked to me, but I listened when he sometimes talked to others, thereby surreptitiously gleaning details of a fairly colourful past life.

Strafings by Stukas on remote French beaches, the roar of hell exposed as Monty unleashed hitherto unimaginable firepower at El Alamein, grisly adventures on the Burma Railway, up to his balls in leech-infested swamp with a knife clenched between his jaws, how the Gurkhas were, to a man, shifty little bastards, how the Empire had gone down the tubes with such staggering rapidity due to limp-wristed ponces of politicians giving the fuzzie-wuzzies far too much say about things that they didn't understand anyway, and how National Service should be brought back and the streets cleared of pimply-faced glue-sniffing little cunts wearing baseball caps back to front who had never done a day's work in their lives. The usual bollocks.

Then there was George, an alcoholic social worker who was obsessed by the idea that the ugly subjects used by the Flemish artist Brueghel in his studies of sixteenth-century peasantry were now all living in Stroke City and following him around the streets.

He also had a recurring dream that all the babies prevented from being born by the Pill had eventually shown up *en masse* in a foul mood demanding some form of redress. I liked George. His employers were puzzled by him, his clients were frightened of him, and his wife had run off with a carpet salesman.

Paddy was a retired funeral director who still wore a neat black suit and sombre tie. His wife had died recently and he regretted that he had been unable to bury her personally. He said it would have made all the difference and asked me how I would like to be buried by strangers. I could only reply that it was something to which I had never given a great deal of thought.

Humpy Danny occupied a corner of his own. Small in stature and with the face of a weasel, he was permanently grouchy and, not surprisingly, did not care to respond to his nickname, due to the fact that he was a hunchback. 'Hunchback' is a cruel, medieval-sounding word but there appeared no alternative way to describe his infirmity. Nor did anyone ever go to much trouble to seek one out.

He was a sad, lonely figure, reminded daily of his plight by the unattractive native Northern Irish habit of referring openly, in an indelicate manner, to imperfections in an individual's physical make-up.

A visually impaired friend of mine never really warmed to the nickname he had been allocated by his peers. People called him Blindy . . .

Humpy Danny was tetchy yet stoical, but could be pushed too far, as he was on one occasion when a fellow drinker suggested he join the Parachute Regiment since, in terms of equipment, he seemed already halfway there.

He drank heavily and needed every drop of it.

Oliver was a defrocked church organist who once had enjoyed almost celebrity status throughout the parish in which he laboured. His fall from grace was rumoured to have been the outcome of some unpleasantness involving boys in a belfry . . . but nobody ever talked about that.

He was urbane, erudite and not a little sinister. He and I had things in common. I once told him how I had lost my religion.

As a twelve-year-old I had been a member of a church choir which serviced a prominent cathedral. My fellow choristers and I were usually located on a high balcony which protruded from the back wall of the church. This meant that the organist/leader of the choir had to perform with his back to the altar, which was situated at the opposite end of the building.

The main entrance to the cathedral was directly below us and therefore out of sight. When a particular service called for the local bishop to enter in some splendour, we were required to sing the celebratory hymn 'Ecce Sacerdos', which I quickly realised was the bishop's 'signature' tune. When it was time for his glorious entry, the worker-bee priest at the altar, seemingly involved in communication with the Higher One, was, in fact, informing the organist via a series of complicated hand signals (observed through the wing mirrors on the organ) of the progress of the bishop.

When the proper psychological moment arrived to give the bishop's entry maximum clout, a signal was made, the organ blared majestically, and we lustily sang our hearts out for the benefit of the fat prelate who strode airily down the aisle whilst the lumpenproletariat clamoured to clutch the hem of his raiment.

In a flash I realised that this wasn't religion at all. It was showbusiness.

I confessed to Oliver that this was a turning point in my life and I regarded myself fortunate indeed to have recognised the reality of godly worship before I was tainted fatally by religious fervour.

He replied only that he was surprised it had taken me so long to figure it out.

It was Oliver who told the clientele about archaeopteryx.

It came out of nowhere.

It started when he turned to Humpy Danny and asked, 'Do you have a budgie?'

Humpy Danny fidgeted and looked startled. But after a short period of time mulling the question over in his mind lest it contain the seed of a personal insult, he deemed it safe to reply. 'Yes,' he said. 'As a matter of fact, I do.'

'Thought so. Well, next time you look at your budgerigar,' Oliver said, 'think dinosaur.'

He settled back on his stool and clasped his hands over his sumptuous belly.

'Science has proven beyond any reasonable doubt that all birds are descended from a single source, much the same way as the origin of man can be traced to the hominids, or apes to you, unless of course you subscribe to one or other of the Creationist theories, which, I'm sure, as a sensible man, you don't.'

Oliver had now engaged the attention of the entire slack-jawed bar.

'In the case of birds,' he continued, 'that common ancestor was archaeopteryx, the first winged, feather-driven, flighted dinosaur; not to be confused with nefarious inferior gliding or skin-flapping aerial creatures of the age, such as the popular pterodactyl. We're talking Jurassic period here,' he sniffed importantly. 'As archaeopteryx developed, more feathers appeared, mobility increased and the bones of the flighted beast hollowed out, rendering the creature more aero-dynamically sound and altogether a more adaptable kettle of fish . . .'

'Load of crap!' muttered Second World War Jack through his pipe.

'Let him speak,' chortled Doomed Social Worker George. 'The man's on a roll.'

'Thank you,' said Oliver Organ. 'So . . . being the only dinosaur aloft and being heavily feathered, therefore insulated, it was equipped to survive whatever great disaster occurred at that unhappy time that wiped the dinosaurs from the face of the earth. Do you follow me, lad?'

'I think so,' said Humpy Danny.

'So, Danny. The dinosaur converted into something else entirely – your actual birds. And the smartest bird of all is the budgie, because it's got you to feed it and take care of it. Were dinosaurs smart or what?'

'So?' said Humpy Danny.

'So?' said Oliver. 'So this. It gives a man heart. It goes to show that all is never lost. Nothing ever goes away, if you know what I mean. Life just . . . transmogrifies. Informed scientific opinion indicates that we may all be wiped out on some future cataclysmic day. The most likely cause of our demise will be the disintegration of the ozone layer, followed by a steep rise in temperature. The whole world will turn into featureless desert and human life as we know it will cease to be.'

Humpy Danny was confused. 'But aren't you arguing against your own theory? What's your point? According to you, life will go on in some other form.'

'Yes,' said Oliver, 'but some of us will have certain advantageous physical characteristics that will enable those who carry our genes to survive in a hostile environment.'

Humpy Danny didn't see it coming.

Neither did I.

'Your progeny, Danny, will survive. In a Doomsday situation I have high hopes for your line in a parched world. Your descendants are more likely than those of anyone here to evolve into camels!'

Oliver leaned back and lit a celebratory pipe.

Danny's hunched back seemed to twitch involuntarily.

The brothers looked anxiously at each other.

At some preordained signal that I failed to catch, one of them lifted the broom to sweep the floor whilst the other stood on a chair and changed a light bulb that looked perfectly functional to me.

Time, gentlemen, please.

ANORAKS AND
ANACHRONISMS

IT WAS MAY 1992, and I found myself once more standing underneath Eric Gill's sculpture of the boy god Ariel that stares disdainfully over the heads of those poised to pass through the doors of Broadcasting House in London. I was surprised to be there, convinced I had blown my chance of any kind of upward mobility by daring to disagree with the Controller of Radio 2.

A year later, and here I was, toeing the threshold of Radio 4, of all places.

I had hitherto not held any strong opinions about Radio 4, idly regarding it as the exclusive preserve of a small band of harmless souls who had never really recovered fully from a university education. The kind of people who didn't understand why other people didn't like them.

I had been asked to present an edition of a Radio 4 programme called *Pick of the Week*, filling in for the regular presenter, who had taken a week off for rest and recreation.

Apparently I had been chosen because of a short voice-piece I had been asked to do for another programme altogether. This involved relating episodes from a previous life when I had been gainfully employed in an Irish showband travelling the length and breadth of the Old Sod playing bad music we didn't like for people who didn't want to listen to us. This chronicling of a character-forming occupation, involving as it did heavy drinking and the frequent attempted

deflowering of the innocent female Irish peasantry by flash-
suited, insincere showbusiness casualties like myself, was
perceived to have some merit, and word of it had reached the
ears of influential people. I was somewhat surprised at this, as
my method of rough reportage seemed at odds with the
general tenor of the usual fare favoured by the station.

This was before I discovered that the people behind the
scenes at Radio 4, the producers, researchers etc., are much
more civilised, open and normal than most of the presenters,
or indeed most of what is known as the network's 'hard-core'
listening audience.

But all this was ahead of me as I entered the foyer of the
fabled building. Wholesome pink faces stared down upon me
from the portraits on the walls. I was pierced by the steely
smile of Sue Lawley, intimidated by John Humphrys' gimlet
gaze, beheld the rapidly balding head of Ken Bruce and
marvelled at Gloria Hunniford's gleaming teeth. I felt the
phantom hand of Lord Reith upon my shoulder, but the hand
was soon swiftly withdrawn when I stepped into a lift to find
that among my fellow passengers was the then Radio 1 DJ
Danny Baker, accompanied by a man with bulging eyes and a
bad wig.

Eavesdropping whilst busily examining my ragged finger-
nails, I heard Baker refer to an obviously absent colleague as a
'facking KANT!'.

This is the place for me, I thought. Not in the building two
minutes and already I hear casual talk of German
philosophers.

Pick of the Week was usually recorded on a Friday evening,
and I was required to clock in on a Tuesday, spending from
then until Friday listening to assorted meritorious bits of the
previous week's radio output from across the land.

The offices occupied by the programme's staff had a
pleasant and faintly donnish atmosphere, not yet pruned
down, computerised or terrorised by the Birtian pogroms that
were to come later.

Darkly dressed slim women floated by, flashing egregious

smiles, or sat with hunched backs and furrowed brows over electric typewriters whilst I waded through my pile of cassette copies of radio programmes purporting to be the best broadcasting that the English language had to offer the world during the course of that particular week.

I found most of the material fairly boring, except for a stimulating interpretation of Pinter's *No Man's Land* by two doughty theatrical knights. One of them was Dirk Bogarde; the other wasn't. There was a dark documentary about heavy drinking and casual fornication in darkest Glasgow called *Jason and the Thunderbird* (Jason being the louche, dole-signing Lothario of the piece, who preyed upon married women, and Thunderbird a brand of cheap, potent wine favoured by the Scottish lumpenproletariat).

This could be worse, I thought. This is good stuff. I'm on top of this.

I then picked up a copy of a programme from something called *File on 4*.

File on 4 was a series I hadn't heard of before, and this particular edition was about theatrical agents and their shady dealings with members of the acting profession.

I thought it hilarious. A stunningly well-written, beautifully observed comedy, complete with bland, pompous narrator whose deadpan, humourless commentary perfectly ignored the surreality of preposterous tales told of unsecured pantomime roles, precious actors whingeing over petty imagined slights, slimy agents (usually called Solly) disappearing overnight clutching paper bags bursting with ten-pound notes. Every ridiculous showbusiness stereotype was ruthlessly lampooned in what I thought was a genuine comedic *tour-de-force* ... a perfect parody of the type of vacant documentary that used to be made by the BBC in the fifties before they discovered that there were people alive out there. Eat your heart out, Peter Sellers.

I couldn't wait to share my discovery. But I was alone in the office at the time.

Eventually the programme's production assistant returned

from lunch. She was wispily beautiful, with long shining hair and soft lips. I fancied her a great deal.

'You wanna listen to this!' I enthused. 'This is the funniest thing I've ever heard in my life! It's a masterpiece.'

I rushed to the cassette player and excitedly rewound the tape.

'What's the programme?' she enquired enthusiastically, adjusting her admirably short skirt.

'Something called *File on 4*,' I blurted breathlessly. 'Heard of it?'

'*File on 4*?' she repeated, seemingly perplexed.

'Yeah,' I said. 'Have you heard it before? Who are the writers? They're brilliant.'

'Are you certain it's *File on 4*? And it's a comedy piece?'

'Yes.'

'They don't usually do that sort of thing.'

'Just listen to it.'

I put the tape on.

She sat throughout with a stony face whilst I whooped uncontrollably.

The tape came to an end.

'I don't know how to tell you this,' she said, after a grim pause, 'except to say that it's not meant to be funny. It's a straight documentary.'

'Are you serious?' I asked.

'Yes.'

'It couldn't possibly be! It's pure Monty Python. How can it be serious?'

'It is. Would you like to ring their office and ask if it's meant to be funny? That's the sort of thing I normally do, but in this case I would prefer it if you made the call yourself.'

She pursed her red lips.

'No,' I said. 'Let the hare sit.'

'Pardon me?' she said.

'It's an Irish expression. Forget it.'

This was evidence of a possibly insurmountable cultural gap. I should have known then that Radio 4 was not to be the place for me. *File on 4* was a harbinger of something worse to come.

And I hadn't even heard *The Moral Maze* yet.

Apart from this initial blip, things went reasonably well. I listened to all the tapes and cobbled together a programme by means of intense bursts of feverish work sandwiched between my main activity, which consisted of wandering the corridors of the BBC in search of interesting things to look at.

I stalked the premises like a bird-watcher, haunting the BBC canteen for long periods, nursing damaging cups of coffee and eavesdropping the conversation of the likes of Craig Charles (*Red Dwarf*!), who seemed quite agitated about the quality of some script or other. He was wearing an old tweed overcoat that looked freshly out of Oxfam and was delightfully scruffy. I liked him immediately. The man with him looked like a bank clerk. Probably a producer. I listened intently.

'It's a load of rubbish!' exclaimed Charles, waving what looked like a script.

'It's his best shot,' said the bank clerk.

'He'll have to come up with something better than this.'

'That's the best he can do.'

'Never!'

'Believe me.'

They lapsed into silence. I had to stop myself from asking them to argue some more. But they wouldn't.

I directed a confused, salad-toting Richard Todd (*Dambusters*!) towards the mayonnaise and caught Juliet Stevenson's (*Truly, Madly, Deeply*!) eye in the lift.

A harassed Michael Buerk (Ethiopian famine!) once knocked me sideways in a corridor when he and I collided at a blind sharp corner, the impact causing him to drop the sheaf of papers he was desperately clutching. He hurriedly picked them up, muttering under his breath.

He didn't see me at all.

White men can take it.

I drank in the atmosphere of the BBC. There is nothing else quite like it. An air of calm intelligence tempered by otherworldly politeness and an incongruent fussiness.

I fingered obscure books in the BBC library. Learned treatises on the Crazy Gang, Donald Peer's autobiography, the Definitive Victor Sylvester, the Essential Liberace . . . dog-eared and well-thumbed.

I peeped hesitantly into the offices of *Woman's Hour* and savoured the air of efficiency, equality and easy dignity, as befits an institution that bears the White Woman's Burden of articulating the hopes, dreams and fantasies of feminine Middle England.

I was frightened by the determined masculinity and the reek of an intolerable workload that emanates from the *Today* headquarters. Players all. Men who are ahead of the posse at all times. It seems impossible that smoking is not permitted here. It should be mandatory. The place is crying out for good cigars and snifters of brandy.

I roamed at will, examining wall-frames containing obscure Certificates of Excellence from Poland, photographs of John Peel in Moscow, and Ken Dodd, equipped with tickling stick, standing precariously on a Blackpool Pier rail.

I was a fan . . . an anorak.

I know that now.

My *Pick of the Week* seemed to be received favourably enough, and at a later date, I was contacted by a friendly BBC producer who invited me to meet with him to discuss the possibility of doing a short series, the general content of which he suggested I might care to think about in the mean time.

When the day came for us to put our heads together, I, of course, hadn't thought about it at all.

We repaired for lunch to a small restaurant in Great Portland Street staffed by friendly Italians with cold eyes, and over fettucine and the like, we kicked some ideas around. Fresh ideas for radio programmes are hard to come by, and after I suggested the usual non-starter rubbish such as

travelling the country with a circus, going 'bush' in Cardboard City with a hidden microphone, a day in the life of a
dodgy massage parlour, or real life behind the scenes on the
Orient Express, we fell silent.

I explained that I didn't really want to do a series of
programmes interviewing people.

When he enquired why, I revealed that I didn't really want
to talk to anybody at all. For reasons that I didn't quite
understand. Maybe something anti-social.

That settled, we forgot about talking about radio, ordered
more wine and set about enjoying our lunch.

We relaxed.

Small talk began.

'How are things at home in Northern Ireland?' he said.
'Looks bad in the papers.'

'You should never believe anything you read about
Northern Ireland in the newspapers,' I replied.

'Really?' he said.

'Yes, because things in Northern Ireland are always so
much worse. Can you imagine a sinking ship crewed by rats
who are prepared to go down with it?'

'That's a difficult one.'

'Well, it's the closest analogy I can think of.'

'You poor man.'

'It's simple. Two communities straining at the leash,
waiting to tear the other's throats out. But apart from that,
everything is OK.'

'OK?'

'Yes, within their own communities people in Northern
Ireland are happy and well adjusted . . . models of tolerance.'

'That doesn't add up.'

'Where else would you find an alcoholic terrorist dwarf?'

'A what?'

'An alcoholic terrorist dwarf,' I replied, with some
satisfaction.

I told him about Stroke City and some of its peculiarities.
I told him about the sign hanging over a city-centre

restaurant that proudly proclaimed '24-HOUR CAFÉ . . . OPEN 9 to 5'.

I told him about the native of Stroke City who defended himself against a charge of riotous behaviour by testifying that an Army Land Rover had repeatedly reversed into his fist in which he was inadvertently holding an iron bar.

I told him that we had the only five-year-old Norman fort in Europe.

I told him about another native of Stroke City who, when searched by the Army, was discovered to have in his trouser pocket a small primed bomb, which, had it exploded, would have killed everyone within a ten-yard radius, including himself. He claimed no prior knowledge of its existence and testified that he could only assume someone had put it there as a practical joke.

I told him that it was a city comprised of extremely tightly knit communities fashioned by traditional loyalties and long-term need, where people looked after each other and were emotional about it. A good place, where no one was left out in the cold or forced to fend for themselves.

I told him it was a city where a dwarf's flat could be raided by the Army and found to contain a Russian surface-to-air rocket launcher capable of bringing down the biggest helicopter extant.

I explained that in this modern world where an average dwarf would have some difficulty leading a normal life unconnected with showbusiness, it was, in some ways, comforting to know that this tiny individual was so integrated into the community that he had gained the complete confidence of, and was acceptable to a lethal, dedicated paramilitary organisation.

Nor was it the case that he was merely exploited by the paramilitaries on the premise that, being a dwarf and therefore distinctive, he would never be suspected by the authorities of working actively towards the destruction of the State.

No. He had been a visible presence during the nascent days of the 'Troubles'.

In the early seventies there was an area of Stroke City known as 'Free Derry' (i.e. the Bogside) in which, for a period of time, no member of the security forces dared set foot. This created a window of opportunity for men stout and true to come forward and declare themselves local custodians of public order, 'vigilantes', in fact, most of whom would later progress to something more sinister.

Duties included monitoring traffic, appearing to keep a lid on petty crime (there's a term for that in Northern Ireland – ODC – Ordinary Decent Crime, as opposed to terrorism) and generally repelling boarders.

These men were armed (after a fashion) and, crucially, hooded, no doubt figuring that anonymity would command respect and create not a little fear. Unfortunately, in a community where everybody knows everybody else, if a vigilante is just under three feet six inches tall, wearing a hood is not exactly perfect as a means of concealing one's identity. Our small friend soon realised this, at considerable cost to his dignity, but persevered in the bullish hope that one fine day he would not be recognised.

It is to the eternal credit of those around him that he was not discouraged from this line of work.

From an unlikely source, that, in my book, is humanity at its best.

With the passage of time, the little fellow developed a drink problem, and was finally caught in possession of arms and sentenced to a ten-year stretch, during which, I am told, he suffered untold agonies and gross humiliation in communal prison showers.

Taking the long view, sometimes it's not such a good idea to get to piss with the big boys.

My BBC producer friend listened intently, raised a glass and announced:

'That's it! We have the theme of our series. Let's call it *Surviving in Stroke City!*'

'All right!' said I.

Anyway, I'd always had a thing about dwarves.

Years ago, I befriended a young lady dwarf (if that's not politically incorrect) in Belfast. She was bubbly, intelligent and had the most beautiful smile I had ever seen.

I lost contact for a couple of years until one night she walked into a club in Belfast.

I was standing alone at the bar, drinking a small Bush. She was with non-vertically challenged friends and occasionally cast puzzled glances in my direction. I wanted to go over and say hello but realised with horror that I had completely forgotten her name and shamefully avoided her eye.

She took it upon herself to make the first move. She came over, smiled a beatific smile and I gladly but guiltily bent down to hug her.

'Gerry, why didn't you come over and join us? Why are you standing there on your own?' she chirped.

'It's great to see you, luv,' I said. 'To tell you the truth, I was embarrassed because, for some reason, I have totally forgotten your name, and I was biding my time, trying to remember. Isn't that stupid of me?'

I thought it better to display honesty.

She laughed gaily.

'Don't be silly. I'm Judy . . . remember? I was worried for a moment. I thought you didn't recognise me.'

I thought that was nice.

I admired her pluck.

For a person who stood out from the herd, this town was no place to be on a Saturday night.

DRUNKEN DWARVES AND
PRIVATE THOUGHTS

BELFAST IS A hard, cruel town inhabited by the best and worst people ever to enter into this bounteous world, people who, unfortunately, due to bad planning on the part of whatever passes for a Creator, happen to live next door to each other.

It takes a special breed to see nothing unusual in being proud of having built the *Titanic*, and to be fair, it is true to say that without the special dedication and supreme craftsmanship of the Belfast ship-yard worker, the *Titanic* wouldn't be where she is today.

The people possess a flint-like sense of humour that is an echo of hard times, and recent lethal times are the result of a heady mix of Irish fecklessness and unforgiving Scottish Calvinism; an amalgam of light-hearted tolerance and a 'bleak bowler-hatted refusal of the inevitable'.

It's an interesting place.

The Europa Hotel in Belfast is the most bombed hotel in the world, but you'd never guess that, observing the cheeky, smiling faces of the wise-cracking barmen who minister to the incessant demands for drink from the patrons of the front downstairs bar.

For a four-star hotel, the clientele is surprisingly varied; captains of industry mix freely with human pond-life.

Business is brisk due to the imminent prospect of Christmas, and I'm doing what I have done every Thursday night for the past couple of weeks. I'm drinking with the dwarves.

There are six of them, in high spirits, fresh from performing with Snow White in the ornate Victorian theatre across the street which is, as always, the venue for the year's festive pantomime.

These are worldly dwarves, and manage regularly to consume between them a very large number of pints of Guinness, to the extent that I can't help but worry about where this great amount of black liquid can possibly be going.

My worries prove irrelevant as the drinking accelerates and the little men show no sign of easing up or, indeed, being in any way adversely affected. They seem to just about hit their stride round about the time my head begins to spin.

I am, however, supremely confident in my ability to maintain, and find myself wondering what the other denizens of the bar will make of the sight of a well-known and frequently derided local radio and television personality slumped on a bar stool with three pissed dwarves on either side of him.

There should be seven, of course, but I know better than to suggest that the missing one might be Grumpy.

Too obvious . . . disrespectful, too.

I met my dwarves through the Belfast Snow White.

We all hit it off instantly.

They liked my stories.

I told them about my experiences behind the scenes at Disneyland, California, where I was sent to make a stupid radio programme.

In a staff recreation area 'backstage' (as Disneypeople say) a man wearing a gun prevented me from taking a photograph of one of their in-house Mickey Mouses (Mice?), who had taken his head off and placed it on a table in front of him as a prelude to lighting a very large cigar, which he proceeded to enjoy with his two great black mouse feet perched contentedly on a highish stool. Didn't see any harm in the photograph itself. A little Disneyland *vérité*.

The security guards thought differently.

I received a caution.

They also liked my only Snow White story. During the same trip to Disneyland, I was forced to seek out their user-friendly fairytale heroine to ask her the kind of stupid questions I knew she'd be sick of answering.

When I located her, she was surrounded by small, noisy Californian children who were remarkably persistent in their enthusiastic attempts to attract her attention. These were children like no other children I had ever encountered. Californian children differ from all other children in the world in that they have honed the business of being a child to such a fine art that there is no other way to describe them other than as Professional Children.

Snow White held her ground gamely, all the while smiling sweetly, her heavily made-up alabaster face and severe black wig looking strangely menacing in the relentless Californian sun.

I tried to separate her from the pack for the purpose of recording my pointless interview.

Children clawed cruelly at her billowing dress.

'Hey, Snow White, I'm Rick!'

'Hello, Rick! What a nice little boy you are!'

'Hi! Snow White! I'm Bob. Willya sign this?'

A tiny blond cretin held up a crumpled bus ticket for her attention; the cue for other ragged pieces of paper to be thrust forward.

She managed to tear herself away politely from all except one sun-blest brat who refused to be shaken off.

Snow White leaned towards him, baring her teeth in a talk-show-host smile, and whispered:

'Fuck off, sonny, or you'll feel the point of my boot up your ass!'

I fell in love with her immediately.

The look on the child's face was alone worth the price of admission.

The dwarves chuckled darkly at this. They're well used to

the seamy side. Comes with the territory.

They ordered more Guinness.

I don't know why I like the dwarves so much. I suppose it is their happy fatalism.

I recognise this as the attitude adopted by most thinking people who have to live in Northern Ireland. The sensitive souls usually emigrate, leaving behind only the lazy, the ignorant and the physically very strong.

As I sit unsteadily on my bar stool, peering above the over-large heads of the carousing dwarves, I see a fairly representative cross-section of Northern Ireland life squirming and jostling through another night's drinking.

A defeated five-piece band is playing in a corner of the room. At the keyboard of a small electric piano, a fat woman with unseeing eyes is playing wrong chords behind a singer who doesn't know the difference.

He gazes at the ceiling whilst howling, 'I left my heart in San Francisco', not realising that he is too old to wear tight Levi jeans, especially when they have a knife-edge crease.

I recognise his face.

He used to be famous in the old show-band days when people knew no better. He hasn't been told that those days are now gone and, sadly, still retains the affected air and raffish old-fashioned mannerisms of a man who is accustomed to people staring at him admiringly.

They don't, of course.

They are too busy watching a tall, bald man who is dancing with an invisible partner near the door. He glides effortlessly between the tables wearing a ballroom dancer's smirk, oblivious to the muttered threats from some of the seedier elements.

The drummer, a bored, long-faced, thin man with flaking skin, ends the song with a tired snare-drum roll that sounds like a rat running for its life across a tin roof, and the lone dancer raises his left hand in traditional homage to the band whilst his right arm remains affectionately draped over the imaginary shoulders of his non-existent partner, whom he immediately thanks audibly and graciously before striding elegantly through the front door and back into the night.

Standing beside the third dwarf on my extreme left is a quality-broadsheet English journalist engaged in conversation with a man who is proud of the 'Troubles'. There are many of these people to be found in Belfast. Men whose lives are enriched by the idea of corruption, torture, mayhem and sudden death. Men whose life's work is exaggerating to English journalists. No horror story too grim that doesn't play better with a little embellishment.

This particular journalist stands awkwardly at the bar, adopting the posture of a man at a cocktail party who is ill at ease yet striving to get on top of the evening. His companion looks like a man who has spent too much time in public libraries – faded moth-eaten suit, traces of cigarette ash on front of jacket, grubby white shirt, tie askew, two-day growth on chin but obviously a man with a point of view.

'So, what's the answer?' asks the journalist.

'There is no answer,' replies his drinking partner, 'and never will be because people are asking the wrong question.'

'What is the correct question then?'

'Instead of asking why we can't get on with each other here, people should be asking why democracy doesn't work here.'

'Isn't that the same thing?'

'No, it's not, so it's not. People are afraid to utter the unutterable. There's something ugly going on here that so-called civilised people will not face. Civilised people insist on believing that the majority of voters in a well-educated, relatively healthy population of a West European democracy will automatically choose a course that will be mainly acceptable to all. That's the nature of democratic society. That's the rock upon which the notion of freedom firmly stands. That's your Pax Britannica so it is. Northern Ireland is ungovernable because in the English corridors of power, they know that the majority of voters here will always vote for people who will want to sink the ship with the probable loss of all hands. English politicians know this, but they can't ever admit it because they can't be heard to say that democracy doesn't work in a sizeable part of the United Kingdom. It's more than their jobs are worth, so it is. If Hitler was dug up, revived and put forward as a candidate in an election to choose the Prime Minister of Ulster and ran on a manifesto of killing every first-born child and hanging everyone he didn't like the look of, he'd get in on a landslide . . . so he would.' Excited now, he grasps his pint with a delicate hand and gulps it down.

'So, the answer is that there is no answer,' says the journalist.

'Yes, there is an answer. I think the people in this country who don't believe in democracy should be taken out and SHAT!'

I think, he's right, you know, except maybe for the last bit.

One of the dwarves is listing to starboard. Our small group is seated on fairly high bar stools and, should the small man topple, the consequences could be fatal. I take remedial measures and gently right him to the perpendicular, for which act of foresight he thanks me.

A TV set flickers in the corner. Politicians again. More cheap, power-hungry bastards. A local programme. The same red faces fume and splutter, seemingly all talking at once. I say seemingly, because the sound is turned off. It makes no difference. The clientele have heard it all before. The usual game of defending the indefensible by means of selected quotes from the Old Testament. The unspeakable haranguing the unelectable.

A few solitary souls stare dully at the screen, their mouths set in cynical grins.

Oh, of course it's regrettable that early one morning a woman turned up for work at a local newsagent's and, as she was opening the shop, three men jumped out of a car, doused her with petrol and set her alight.

Oh, of course it's unfortunate that elected politicians speak openly of ethnic cleansing in a deliberate attempt to prise open the hooded eyes of the brute that traditionally lurks within the souls of many of their constituents.

Oh, of course it's a shame that politically motivated bands of bullet-headed thugs roam the streets with ugliness on their minds.

Oh, of course it's wrong that half-humans energised by half-truths and misinformation burst into people's homes in the middle of the night and bludgeon their sleepy victims to death with baseball bats.

Maybe this is what Bosnia was like before we got to hear about it. But that's silly talk. That's a foreign country far away, full of weirdos and not a bit like here.

We're part of Great Britain, for fuck's sake!

It could never happen here.

This is the cradle of democracy.

Somebody would stop it.

Wouldn't they?

One of the dwarves was last seen reeling out of control towards the Gents' and has failed to return after what has been deemed a more than reasonable timespan. Another has been dispatched to assess the seriousness of his condition.

A clutch of businessmen gather at the end of the bar, slapping each other's backs and cackling too loudly at jokes that aren't funny.

Pink, healthy, unlived-in, piggy faces contort with laughter whilst their eyes remain watchful. They circle round a central figure who's quieter than the rest and whose suit is noticeably less wrinkled, the mark of a man obviously higher up the corporate pecking order.

The others perform the Businessman's Courtship Ritual – left hand thrust deeply in trouser pocket audibly jangling change, right hand gripping glass against white-shirted chest. The body adopts a ramrod posture, weight shifts regularly from one foot to the other in a nifty little dance of deference. The whole group sways like a drifting clump of seaweed. All have schoolboy haircuts and all are on their best behaviour.

The man with the unwrinkled suit is, I deduce, a born-again Christian or something similarly ascetic. Apart from the fact that no one is drinking alcohol, a young woman with big tits sways past the group on her way to the loo, but not one of them checks out her arse when she passes.

The concentration on making a good impression is obvious. Be focused.

Ring-fence your objectives.

Copper-fasten that promotion.

My mind starts to drift.

One of the dwarves is dressed in miniature leathers and explains to me that he rides a Harley-Davidson because he loves the freedom of the open road and the feel of the wind in his hair. I am having a little trouble with this and am trying to figure out a way to ask him delicately whether or not his Harley is the whole Hog when I am interrupted by a sudden commotion at the door. A number of swarthy men are attempting to gain entrance to this place of entertainment but are being repelled by what Americans now refer to as admission consultants.

A heavily set barman darts swiftly from his post at the pumps to offer the bouncers assistance. By the look in his eyes he's hoping for trouble, but tonight, serious trouble is not to be.

Heated words ensue, but after some minor, powder-puff scuffling the situation is resolved. The refused party grumble loudly and melt away into the night.

The disappointed barman returns with a flushed face. 'Fuckin' tinkers,' he mutters in our general direction.

Ah, I see . . . The residue of a tinker wedding as it turns out . . . in search of that one last drink. The last remnants of the old ways, 'Travelling People' I suppose we have to call them now, rejected but resolute free spirits in the new, increasingly corporate Ireland.

One of the dwarves is English. 'Romany gypsies?' he asks.

'No,' say I. 'Real tinkers. The progeny of those dispossessed during the Great Famine. Black '47. The descendants of those who hadn't the wit or the money to go to America . . . brutally run off their land by money-grabbing bastards from your own country. Condemned to wander rootless like the Children of Israel. There's plenty of them about still, back pockets full of twenty-pound notes, no use for banks, driving new Volvos, gambling, drinking and selling carpets. But they can't settle. They're wild and the wanderlust is in them.'

I decide to tell the dwarves about Pecker Dunne. I know they will like him.

Pecker Dunne claimed to be the last of the genuine Travelling People. He played the banjo spectacularly well and wrote songs about the travelling life. Born on the road and domiciled permanently in a rickety horse-drawn caravan, he was never happy unless mobile. The crunch of iron-clad wheels upon gravel.

He was discovered by a music scout and cajoled into a recording studio where he laid down part of his self-penned idiosyncratic repertoire. As a direct result Pecker found himself with a record in the Irish pop charts.

This unexpected stroke of good fortune necessitated personal appearances – gigs, touring; nothing unusual for him, of course. Happy days, he thought. Except for one small thing which he found difficult.

He was expected to be nice to people.

He was a huge, ill-proportioned man. No part of his body appeared to belong to the whole. Large square head, heavily dented as a result of numerous fist fights, barrel chest tapering abruptly to an almost puny waist, comically over-sized feet and dangling ape-like arms that rippled with muscles. It was said that he once carried a full-grown horse for two miles without any of its hooves ever touching the ground.

He was a gentle soul if he liked you. Difficult if he didn't.

I was a member of his short-lived backing band.

He was peculiar in that he bore grudges against geo-graphical locations. It wasn't that he didn't like people. He didn't like people who lived in particular places.

The dwarves nod.

Maybe they understand Pecker's thought processes.

One night we were due to appear at a dance hall in a town in Co. Cork called Macroom. I found Pecker Dunne wandering about after dark outside the hall, looking around the bushes for something he had lost. I offered assistance. He darted suddenly to the left, snatched something from the grass, stuffed it inside his baggy shirt, and waved me away.

'Never moind. Oi've bin here before,' he grunted, cryptically.

I thought no more about it but couldn't help but notice that when he joined us later on stage, his shirt bulged ominously.

Due to his undeniably rough sex-appeal, the fans, mostly female, were gathered fifteen deep in front of the stage waiting for him to sing. But Pecker's heart didn't seem to be in it and I wasn't at all surprised to hear him stop midway through his first song. The band gradually ground to a halt in his wake.

There was a menacing silence and I knew instinctively that something bad was going to happen.

Pecker reached inside his shirt and pulled out a dead rat.

He held the rat over his head. It was not a pretty sight and was clearly at an advanced stage of putrefaction.

He bellowed wildly and loudly into the microphone.

'Oi've bin here before and by Jazus it gives me little pleasure to be back again after the way yez treated me the last toime. This is what I think of yez!'

He unleashed a blood-curdling yell and flung the rotting rodent into the middle of a ruck of females.

It was the first time I had witnessed the spectacle of a rat bursting.

I do not wish to see anything like that again.

Pecker Dunne, hands on hips, surveyed the havoc and triumphantly exited stage left.

Needless to say, this is not the showbusiness way.

At other times he needed no grudge against a place to behave strangely.

One Saturday night at the Old Shieling Hotel in Dublin, the band was quietly pleased to witness old Pecker going down a treat. The night came to a successful conclusion and encores were demanded by an audience who gave us the honour of a standing ovation, not a thing we were accustomed to.

The clamour for more bawdy songs increased, and of course, Pecker Dunne did not react as any normal person would. Grabbing the microphone, he screamed: 'What do yez want, ya bastards! Do yez want blood? Wha?'

The audience paused, not accustomed to being called 'bastards' by the star act.

Then, recovering and going along with the banter, they good-naturedly screamed back, 'Yes!'

At this positive response, Pecker produced a cut-throat razor.

'Yez want blood. I'll give yez all the blood yez want,' he hissed.

Slowly he opened the razor and, leering madly at the audience, drew the glistening blade firmly across his naked chest. Blood spurted from his bare torso, spattered the boards of the stage and clotted in the luxuriant thatch of his chest hair.

I felt my stomach heave.

All around were heard cries of alarm and the thud of fainting women's bodies hitting the floor.

There then ensued a general scramble for the exits.

Pecker cried: 'Are yez happy now?'

He gazed happily at the chaos as the gore continued to dribble down the front of his trousers . . .

In time, as you might expect, his public appearances lessened and I never heard much about him again, although somehow I instinctively knew that showbusiness wasn't for him . . . not a man to be found on the golf course with Wogan, Brucie and Tarby.

As I conclude this tale, the dwarves fall silent.

I sense that Pecker Dunne is the man they would like to be.

Eventually, one or two of the dwarves begin to show signs of wear and tear.

Heads begin to nod.
Time to call it a night.

The pubs of central Belfast are emptying and armed police stand silently beside grey Army Land Rovers out of which peer nervous soldiers equipped with impossibly fresh young faces. All around is chaos.

Teenagers puke on their shoes, beer bottles splinter, intoxicated women in short skirts cackle lustily, drunken men mumble gibberish as they slump against gable walls earnestly trying to spear unreachable chips that lie locked in lard in the crevices of vinegar-soaked wrapping paper. Taxi-drivers with fat bellies and sleepy eyes peer knowingly from the cocoons of their cabs. Uneaten hamburgers fly through the air. A foreign tourist stands aghast, surveying the scene from the hotel entrance.

I can tell he is a tourist.

He is wearing real clothes.

An emaciated, unshaven, intoxicated man materialises suddenly behind me, and before I can escape, locks my arm in a vice-like grip.

He spins me roughly around and shoves his face two inches in front of mine.

Blasts of foul breath are transferred directly from his lungs to mine.

'Are you yer man off the TV?' he croaks.

'Yes,' I say, retching imperceptibly.

He leans back unsteadily, sways, almost falls.

'Your show's a load of crap . . . and . . . and . . . you're an ugly bastard!'

He loosens his grip and spins away.

Everyone's a critic . . . these days.

EGO AND THE TUBE

AND INDEED TELEVISION is a load of crap, a medium that makes fools of us all.

There was a time when there were two kinds of television; children's television and TV for grown-ups.

Children's television was different in that everything was explained to the viewer in idiot language whilst the presenters reassured the children, made funny faces, rolled their eyes, jumped up and down, waved their arms and tried generally to keep on top of the child's short attention span.

Television for adults did not require presenters to do this, programme makers assuming that the mature viewer had at least a rudimentary grasp of what was going on and an attention span of more than fifteen seconds.

I can't explain what went wrong, but at some stage in the fairly recent past the distinction between children's TV and grown-ups' TV became so blurred that it is now impossible to tell them apart.

Television has become the exact converse of what had always been believed. As a medium, it is somehow strangely uncomfortable with truth and natural human behaviour. Only lies, flamboyance, insincerity and exaggerated gestures seem to register on it.

I had never thought of becoming a TV talk-show host. It just, well, happened.

I suppose I was doomed from the start, not having the necessary blind ambition married to the natural ruthlessness that is essential if one is to be successful in this line of work. My heart just wasn't in it.

I say this not to award myself praise, but rather to demonstrate my initial innocent ignorance of the Machiavellian nature of the world of television.

It's a wonderful education.

I know now that behind the affable exterior of the average caring talk-show host lies the heart of a killing machine. The Talking Head cannot survive otherwise.

It's a dirty job but everybody wants to do it.

Being a television talk-show host requires other dubious talents that cannot be learnt in the normal way. In addition to the ability to exaggerate physical gestures in a way that looks natural, he also requires a facility for looking relaxed when all around are losing their heads, the possession of an unshiftable smirk, a sluggish metabolism and a reliable method of concealing jangled nerves.

It is a job like no other, staggering in its inanity and almost unbearably pressurised.

When two talk-show hosts get together socially they have a natural rapport that comes of a horrendous shared experience, something akin to that endured by two people who meet at a party and discover that both have survived Auschwitz . . . the horror is mutually understood and rarely discussed.

There are, however, exceptions to the rule.

Once, at some benefit dinner or other, I found myself sitting next to a Talking Head who fronted a similar show on another channel. As we morosely swigged bottles of designer beer and sighed at having to be at this backslapfest at all, he turned suddenly to me.

'What kind of talkback do you get?' he asked.

'Wha?' I replied, slightly surprised at this shop talk.

'Talkback in your ear, during the show. What kind do you get?'

'The usual, I suppose. Disjointed, hysterical. If it gets too bad I take it out of my ear.'

I was referring to the ear-piece worn by TV presenters. This is the only line of communication between the genial host and the production staff behind the scenes – director, producer, soundmen, lighting people, production assistants, researchers and any other of a number of dog's-arses who have a direct line to the brain of the Talking Head who is live on air.

It is, by definition, one-way traffic, as the Talking Head cannot respond to insults, instructions or commands issued other than by a subtle flick of a finger or slight nod of the head, due to his preoccupation with being charming to his guests and looking as though he is in control.

'Mine is getting out of hand. I can't take it any more,' he said.

'Do what I do. Take it out of your ear. That'll shut them up,' I suggested.

'Can't do that. Suppose something goes wrong that I need to know?'

'Fuck them,' I said. 'It's your show. You decide how to handle it.'

He was of the opinion that he was not generally shown proper respect and proceeded to furnish evidence of this.

He explained that it was normally his custom at the end of each show to reach under his chair and produce a previously 'planted' bunch of flowers which he would then present to a deserving member of the studio audience who was celebrating a 115th wedding anniversary or something equally astonishing.

This is an unbeatable, well-tested device, used to provide false evidence that the Talking Head cares about ordinary people and wishes to be fondly regarded as one of them.

One night, however, due to a slight miscalculation on his part, he reached for his blooms prematurely, in the mistaken belief that the show was almost over.

Unfortunately he had forgotten about one last guest, who was patiently waiting in the wings, primed and ready to be shooed on to the killing floor.

'That's a pain in the arse,' I said. 'What did you do?'

'A fella can make a mistake, can't he?' he whined. 'It wasn't the end of the world. Anyway, I soon realised the error of my ways.'

'Talkback, of course?' I suggested, sensing something disturbing.

'Yes.'

'What did they say to you?'

'Now what would your people have said to you in that situation?'

I knew what he wanted to hear.

'Let's see. I think they would have said something like, "Too early, Gerry. Take your time. One more guest to go. No sweat. His name is John Doe",' I lied fluently.

He bristled. 'Yeah, you would expect something along those lines, wouldn't you? A gentle correction and a little encouragement accompanied by some helpful information. After all, I'm only human. I can make a mistake, can't I?'

'Of course you can. We all can. What did they say to you?'

I couldn't wait.

'Well,' he said.

I sensed that he regretted mentioning this in the first place but it was too late to stop now.

I pushed him for more.

'Well, what did they say to you?'

'One of them yelled at me, live!' he said.

'Director?'

'Who else!'

'What did he yell at you?'

'"Not yet, for fuck's sake, you big fat stupid fuckin' bastard."'

His face flushed at the painful recollection.

I waited . . . for effect.

'There's not a lot of information in there, is there?' I said.

Talking Heads like us are not paid large amounts of money because we are particularly good at what we do or particularly talented; we are there because we have mastered the art of not looking nervous . . . the illusion of being in control.

Any wanker can go on television and look nervous.

No man appearing live in front of hundreds of thousands or millions of people is relaxed. The trick is to make people think he is relaxed whilst every nerve in his body is jangling at the thought that one false move, wrong word or stumble at a crucial point may end his career.

There are certain things a man must struggle to avoid.

At all costs, one must control the visibly shaking leg, the trembling hand, the sudden all-enveloping blanket of sweat and, most importantly, the Glassy Stare into the camera. There are two distinct types of Glassy Stare:

GLASSY STARE NUMBER ONE

This is born of pure fear. Quite common, and natural.

One must journey to the animal kingdom for enlightenment.

Picture a rabbit rooted on the white line in the middle of a major road, blinded by the oncoming headlights of a speeding car, and you're almost there.

Better still, consider the eyes of a trapped rat as the bared-fanged snake prepares to lunge, and you have some idea of the phenomenon. It's a primeval, wholesome fear. Nothing to be ashamed of.

But . . .

GLASSY STARE NUMBER TWO

This is a different animal entirely. It has nothing to do with fear. In fact, quite the opposite.

Glassy Stare No. 2 occurs when the hypnotised eyes reveal the vacant soul.

It occurs when the owner gazes in wonderment at the TV camera lens and is so thrilled that people out there are actually watching him that he becomes bewitched and partially paralysed by the turbo-charged boost it gives to his ego. This particular stare is an outward manifestation of the most heinous form of self-idolatry. It cries, 'I have made it! I always knew I would! See! Look at me. Me . . . ! ! !'

Only an expert can distinguish between Glassy Stares Nos. 1 and 2, but those who have acquired the gift of spotting it smile softly when they see No. 2 and speak no more of it, because those who have the misfortune to be afflicted by the all-consuming No. 2 are destined never to lose it.

It is who and what they are.

They are lost, and usually have long and successful careers.

As a mere regional TV talking head, one usually has to deal only with Grade B celebrities. As a rule of thumb, those who are successful commercially, but not particularly good at what they do, are generally aware of their lack of talent and tend to compensate by behaving like shits. Insecure soap stars figure high up the list.

On the other hand those, successful or not, who are good at what they do tend to be reasonable human beings, as they don't usually need to resort to shitdom to be noticed or appreciated.

Alas, this is but a general rule, and there are sad cases of people who are talented, successful, famous, and shits as well. Mercifully, I find them few and far between.

Consequently, when I was in the habit of walking into our production office to find out what was happening, my heart would invariably sink at the sight of otherwise intelligent, productive researchers poring over *Hello!* magazine and other celebrity-orientated publications for the purpose of isolating and contracting who knows what variety of currently popular monster for me to talk and be charming to.

There are other rules of thumb:

1 The Celebrity whom you dread meeting because you think he or she will be a shit is invariably charming and gracious.
2 The Celebrity whom you admire and are looking forward

to meeting will turn out to be a vicious bastard.
3 There are Celebrity shits who are unaware that they are shits. These are difficult to deal with, as no rule of thumb applies.
4 There are Celebrities who are shits in private and angelic in public. These are to be avoided as often as humanly possible. They are the worst kind, causing one to lose faith in the notion of the essential human decency of *Homo sapiens*.
5 Don't ever aspire to Celebrity. It will ruin your life.
6 If you ever do rope a Grade A Celebrity, those around you will always let you down.

Grade A celebrities won't travel to appear on regional talk-shows but sometimes they will permit the regional talk-shows to come to them.

This usually requires a trip to London, where the Talking Head, accompanied by his own pared-down local crew, will be told to appear at, say, the Dorchester Hotel, and join other regional Talking Heads and their crews in an anteroom where all will be processed by the star's harassed PR person.

This person will usually be female and dismissive, treating us minor TV types like plague bacilli.

If the star is a major film hero, we will be told what he or she doesn't want to discuss, which usually encompasses just about everything of any interest.

Everyone will get ten minutes in the presence of the Great One and we must be on our best behaviour lest the star huffs. After all, we are fortunate to be there.

The Talking Head, his director and cameraman will then be exposed to the Presence.

At this moment our own director will invariably let us down. In my experience, our director will be male, about thirty-five years old, and will affect the air of someone who deals with movie stars on a regular basis, which, of course, he doesn't.

Devoid of talent or any sign of proficiency in interpersonal skills, he will force a tight smile and take command of the situation.

This is when the Talking Head must protect himself lest the Presence concludes that he (the Talking Head) is happy with the director's approach and is therefore, by definition, also a wanker.

Take the case of Leslie Nielsen, star of the various *Naked Gun* movies.

Ushered into his aura, I found him a personable chap, and during the course of a preliminary chat whilst the camera was being adjusted, I discovered that we had a mutual ear problem, he being deaf, I marginally less so.

He fished out of each ear what looked to me like orange pips, and explained that these were his revolutionary new hearing aids. I marvelled at their modernity, efficacy and supreme portability.

We were getting on fine until interrupted by my director, who rudely terminated the affable conversation.

'Look, Leslie,' he barked, with all the charm of an SS death-camp guard, 'this is the way it's going to be!'

He then explained in quite unnecessary detail that I would be filmed asking the star questions whilst both of us sat face-to-face on fine armchairs. The fact that we were already doing just that seemed to have escaped his notice.

'And remember, Leslie, this interview will not be seen just in Northern Ireland, but throughout the whole of Ireland!' he barked.

Leslie Nielsen looked at me blankly. Time to step in.

'Now there is no cause for alarm, Leslie,' I said. 'Just remain calm. I know that when you came in here, you thought that this interview was solely for Ulster but now that you know it's for the entire country of Ireland there is no reason to panic.'

Pro that he was, he picked up on it immediately.

'The whole country!' he cried. 'Jesus!'

'Just keep your answers short, concentrate on the questions, and I think we'll get through this thing OK,' I said.

He hesitated. 'I don't know if I can handle this.' He gave a short, low whistle. 'The whole of Ireland!'

The director was alarmed. 'Is there a problem?'

'Let me have a word,' I said soothingly, leading him across the room by the arm. 'I think I can smooth this out.'

Mr Nielsen and I resumed our conversation about hearing aids and then conducted the usual perfunctory celebrity interview. Ending the piece with a little bit of the usual celeb horseplay with golf clubs, we were once again interrupted by the director, who brusquely informed Nielsen that what he was doing could be funnier.

He then explained how the star should readjust his routine to render it more amusing. This master of deadpan comedy calmly followed these instructions whilst I waited in vain for the ground to open and swallow me.

Some people have no sense of shame, nor must aspiring TV talk-show hosts possess anything resembling it.

I have been filmed wearing a dandy dress suit and rakish silk scarf in the glamorous setting of a trendy but grimy London nightclub during a scorching hot summer's day, pretending to quaff champagne with Jackie Collins whilst outside could be heard, very clearly, the clank of dustbins being emptied into revving lorries.

The illusion of glamour is enough.

I have seen and heard things forbidden to ordinary mortals.

I have seen an actress drinking her own piss.

I have seen Gary Glitter without his wig.

I have been shouted at by Bob Geldof.

I have been mesmerised by Nicole Kidman.

Lionel Bart has sung snatches from *Oliver!* to me, waving a badly gashed finger.

I have gotten drunk with the man who used to hand Elvis Presley his scarves on stage.

I have seen an eighty-year-old Stephan Grappelli drink more than half a bottle of Scotch and immediately walk on stage to play the most exquisite, intricate jazz violin without fumbling a note.

I have told a well-known pop singer to go fuck himself.

I have picked up valuable tips by listening to Sacha Distel chatting up young women.

I have played a wobble-board with Rolf Harris.

I have looked Simon Weston straight in the eye.

I have executed a dual pratfall with Norman Wisdom.

I have interrupted Frank Carson and survived.

On a mad whim, I once passionately embraced a pneumatic Miss World and was both surprised and flattered to find that she seemed to quite enjoy it.

I have towered over Adam Faith.

I have interviewed a very old woman who vividly described the expression on her father's face as he gently lowered her from the deck of the sinking *Titanic* into the outstretched arms of her mother who was waiting in a dangling lifeboat.

I have been straight man, fool, aggressive interviewer, sympathetic presence, philanthropist, sycophantic arse-licker, bringer of knowledge and Showbiz Wanker.

It's a full life.

But they don't make celebrities like they used to.

I've only met one person whom I considered to be a real star. You've probably never heard of him.

His name was Ronnie Hawkins . . . 'the Hawk'.

ACCORDIONS AND
CHICKEN WIRE

'LISTEN, SON. IF you join my band, you won't make much money, but you'll get more pussy than Frank Sinatra.'

The words came from the depths of a heavy black beard which was also acting as temporary home to a large, expensive, hand-rolled Havana cigar. Puffs of dense smoke spiralled over an immaculately white stetson perched at a jaunty angle on the bullish head.

A pair of surprisingly small hands were folded daintily across an expanse of protruding white-shirted stomach. The soberly suited figure swung his legs on to a bar stool to reveal a pair of exquisitely crafted snakeskin cowboy boots.

'Whaddya say, son?' the figure said, removing the cigar from his maw and spitting gently but copiously on to the bar-room floor.

I stared blankly back at him.

The year was 1973 and the pair of us were sitting in a rock 'n' roll hang-out called the Nickelodeon on Yonge Street in downtown Toronto. Stevie Wonder's 'Superstition' thundered brassily from the elaborate house sound system, the bass notes mashing our eardrums. The scattered afternoon clientele was made up mainly of ten-dollar hookers, resting strippers, pimps, drug-dealers, burnt-out cases, con-men, gangsters, minor crooks and petty thieves, all of whom were enjoying early-afternoon weak beer poured from communal pitchers provided by a topless French-Canadian waitress of stunning proportions . . . rock 'n' roll heaven.

I was sitting with Ronnie Hawkins, the last and most articulate of the early pioneer rockers.

Born in Huntsville, Arkansas, 'the Hawk' learnt his trade playing the Memphis 'chitlin' starvation circuit using the 'Arkansas credit card' – a siphon, a rubber hose and a five-gallon can. He'd had few commercial hits in the States but rock 'n' roll insiders worshipped him as a god. Bob Dylan and John Lennon regularly sat slack-jawed at his feet as the singer regaled them with tales of the early days touring with Elvis Presley and Jerry Lee Lewis, barnstorming days during the birth in the southern states of what we now know as rock 'n' roll.

Lurid accounts of unbridled debauchery intertwined with epic stories of hell-hole nightclubs dismembered by chainsaws or, indeed, burnt to the ground as a direct result of a shady impresario's failure to pay the Hawk for musical services rendered.

An indefatigable dispenser of folk wisdom, it was the Hawk who first speculated thus: 'Abraham Lincoln said all men are created equal . . . but then he never saw Bo Diddley in the shower.'

He was a master story-teller who lived life to the full. In his early days, he had harboured an ambition to own a Rolls Royce and, eventually, finding himself in the financial position so to do, he proudly entered a car showroom and viewed an exquisite Silver Cloud.

Unfortunately, due to his scruffy appearance in those far-off days, he received short shrift from the sniffy junior salesman. The Hawk repaired quietly to his bank, from which he withdrew $35,000 in one-dollar bills and bundled them into a large brown paper bag.

He re-entered the car showroom toting the bag and again approached the junior salesman.

'Get me the manager,' he demanded.

The young salesman duly obliged.

'How much is that Silver Cloud Rolls Royce?'

'Thirty-five thousand dollars, sir,' the manager replied.

'I'll take it,' said the Hawk, emptying the contents of the bag on to the floor.

'How much does this cocksucker of a salesman usually earn in sales commission?'

'Five per cent,' replied the manager.

The Hawk bent down and scooped up approximately $1,750 from the floor.

'Well, he didn't earn it this time around,' he said. 'I'll take it.'

He stepped into the car and roared off, a swarm of single dollar bills fluttering in his wake.

For months after, the Hawk would occasionally give some wino twenty dollars to go into the same showroom, seek out the hapless junior salesman, and express an interest in buying the most expensive car in the place. The various winos were invariably treated with extreme courtesy.

That's rock 'n' roll star quality.

That same Silver Cloud Rolls Royce, with a hawk in flight emblazoned on each door, now sat outside the Nickelodeon with an unconventionally attired chauffeur lounging in the driver's seat, squinting in the bright sunlight.

Inside, the Hawk was waiting for a reply.

'Yes, I'd love to join the band,' I stuttered.

'OK. You'll wanna know the roools of the band! Well, the roools are that there are no roools save but one. Don't fuck up! Ah don't care what you do. You can drink till your liver ups and growls at you. You can take whatever drugs you want at any time . . . heroin, cocaine, whatever . . . Have fun! And when you come on that stage Ah don't expect you to be sober and Ah don't expect you to be straight. Hell, Ah'm easy to work for! Ah don't care if you come on stage nekkid and Ah don't care if you've just hacked your mother to death with a blunt machete ten minutes before. You can do anything you want any time you want except for one thing. Ah don't want to ever hear no bad notes coming from your guitar. That'll git you fired for shore! All you gotta do is play good and you and Ah'll git along. Welcome aboard and may God protect you, son!'

With that he took his leave, spraying a bluster of bonhomie at the assembled flotsam and jetsam in the bar.

I stared at him in wonder. This was what I had always wanted. An Equal Opportunities employer.

And he was right. There were no rules. There never had been. This was a long way from the dilapidated pub in Stroke City where I had first nervously plucked my guitar for money.

That was a bad time to be young and impressionable.

Marauding sailors of every nationality roamed the streets in a frenzied search for blood and carnal pleasure: crazed Swedes, fearsome Norwegians, small, poisonous Portuguese, loud Brits, screaming Americans, brutal Canadians, combative Danes and the dour Dutch took over Stroke City for a significant proportion of the year, ostensibly taking part in the annual NATO exercises, but in reality engaged in an unofficial mission, the object of which was to loudly seek out and destroy every woman over the age of sixteen.

It was the late fifties and I wasn't much used to this sort of thing, choosing to spend most of the time in my bedroom with a cheap acoustic guitar laboriously learning the chords of hopelessly old-fashioned chestnuts of songs like 'All the Things You Are,' and 'Love is a Many Splendour'd Thing'.

Although I lived in the centre of Stroke City close to the docks, I wasn't much troubled, although regularly comforted, by the smash of bottles in the middle of the night and vile-sounding oaths screamed in a variety of alien tongues.

In addition to the invading hordes there was a community of permanent aliens, whom we would refer to as the 'local Americans', stationed at the permanent naval base on the outskirts of the city – familiar fixtures on the limited social scene.

They were a self-contained community, living within the confines of the base where they had constructed a micro-

America – a source of wonder to the few locals who were granted brief access to this paradise containing manicured lawns with automatic sprinklers, pizzas, Lucky Strike cigarettes, refrigerators, hi-fis, real hamburgers, soda fountains complete with jerk, juke-boxes containing current American hits, good cigars, coffee that didn't make you want to puke, beer that didn't come down your nose, and women in stretch pants with Jayne Mansfield tits. These wonders contrasted vividly with the world which lay outside the starred and striped gates – a dull, sluggish city awash with ill-dressed, spindly-legged, whey-faced, undernourished males dreaming of employment, gathering at mouldy street corners spitting importantly at the pavement, sucking on the grubby remnants of Woodbine dog-ends and subsisting on a hearty diet of spuds, mince, chain-bones, pig's feet and sticky buns.

But even this home from home could not hold some of the wilder Yanks, who roared out of the gates in imported Chryslers and mightily finned Thunderbirds to hit the seedier local pubs in search of a little rough.

Pubs, therefore, held more than the scent of danger.

You know you are in a real pub when you witness, as I once did, the sight of a drunken Portuguese matelot proceeding towards the Gents', unaware that a goodly sized knife was protruding from the small of his back.

The ugly news of this was conveyed to him by means of alarmed cries from casual observers, and only then did he begin to behave like a man who had a knife in his back, i.e., fall to the floor and writhe violently in apparent pain. The way knifed people do in the movies.

I wonder if he lived.

In the midst of such brutality and one-sided affluence, impoverished locals like myself could only look on with the eyes of Bambi, in the grip of a primeval reticence tempered only by innocence.

Music was an escape of sorts, and, on the plus side, some of us didn't look quite as local as others.

Jody certainly didn't fit. His father was a long-gone, black

GI, and his mother an alabaster-faced, flame-haired product of the hills of Donegal. This was a heady mixture of genes. Jody had inherited his father's pigmentation and desperately strove to become an American, an ambitious aspiration for a man who was an illegitimate, black, unemployed Irish Catholic who lived in the Bogside and used the same rough Stroke City accent as the rest of us.

Jody had a good singing voice, not unlike that of his idol, Johnny Mathis, and went to considerable trouble kitting himself out in current American fashion – loafers, white socks, checked red pants, striped blue shirt and loosely hanging cardigan, from the left pocket of which usually peeped a soft pack of cool filter cigarettes.

Sartorially complete, the noble brown head was crowned by a 'flat-top' or 'crew-cut' which he had persuaded a nervous local barber to inflict upon him using as a guide a likeness of the actor Tab Hunter ripped from the pages of an old edition of *Photoplay*.

He had somehow procured what could loosely be described as a cabaret spot, singing in a festering dungeon that we shall name the Wagon Wheel, a notorious hell-hole frequented by card-sharps, lost souls, drunken sailors, wild women and qualified prostitutes.

Jody's talents did not extend to playing the guitar, so I was sequestered to provide musical accompaniment.

It was to be my first 'gig' of any kind, and one for which I feared my Christian Brothers' education had ill prepared me.

Jody's metaphorical carapace was thick. Little deterred him. Not the fierce, drink-fuelled abuse that assailed us as we took the stage, nor the fact that the Americans fell about with laughter when they heard Jody's Stroke City accent. Americans to this day still fall about when they hear black people speak with Irish or British accents. Many find themselves unable to make the required logical leap.

I was terrified. I'd had a word with the proprietor, a devious swine who wore a pasted-on smile whilst he short-changed the baying scum that constituted his clientele.

'Get up and play something, quick,' he hissed. 'Calm the fuckers down.'

Hoarse-throated women were perched high on bar stools (skirts hitched to the limit, baring pock-marked legs and worse), swatting panting sailors with foul words. Occasional pints of Guinness flew across the room, splintering noisily, causing stout-spattered people to rise from their seats and seek redress by means of unarmed combat.

I clutched my guitar like a life-raft and shuffled behind Jody in the corner of the room.

His eyes seemed far away as he slowly reached out to remove the primitive microphone from its stand.

A nasal New York voice rose above the general din:

'Givvus some fuckin' rock 'n' roll, for Crissakes!'

Jody didn't seem to hear him. He was somewhere else where I couldn't reach him.

He smiled dreamily and gently cleared his throat.

In the midst of this chaos and danger he leaned towards me and whispered softly:

'Gimme an A.'

With trembling fingers, I formed the chord of A major and strummed it twice.

At this sound, Jody slowly lit his cool filter, let his right hand dangle and bent his upper body to form the standard New York nightclub casual stoop.

He raised his head sideways towards the microphone, half closed his eyes and slowly opened his mouth to sing.

He sang like some exotic bird.

'Look at me. I'm as helpless as a kitten up a tree.'

Jody had left us. He was in America. Back home where he belonged.

It's 1964 and I find myself somewhere else . . . in an Irish club in Manchester long since demolished for the benefit of all concerned.

I am now a seasoned professional musician. I am twenty years old, a member of the club's resident Irish band, at the wrong end of half a dozen amphetamine tablets, and waiting to take the stage for another hard day's night.

A preceding musical *hors d'oeuvre* is being announced by a round, sweating, carbuncled, hoary-handed compère who grasps the microphone with the not inconsiderable force that he, as a demolition worker by day, has at his disposal.

He thumps the mike viciously to ensure that it is functioning and stiffens formally before shouting:

'Bit o' order now, please, bit o' hush, will yez! On behalf of the committee, please put your hands togedder for Bline Billy Quinn from Ballyconnell. He's here special for yez tonight playing the accordeen. Give 'im a big hand now 'cos he's not only bline, but bline from birth ... Bline from Birth Billy Quinn, come on ...'

Bline Billy Quinn is very blind indeed ... and also very drunk, as is evident from the manner in which he stumbles from the wing of the shoddy stage.

He's a small, hunched man, and bearing his huge accordion with some difficulty, he gropes wildly for the straight-backed chair that has been placed for his benefit in the centre of the performing area.

He plonks himself down heavily and paws the air for the microphone stand, which he eventually locates, lowering its business end in such a manner that the microphone points directly at the vitals of his giant instrument.

No one offers any assistance.

He has now settled. The accordion obscures his entire upper body, revealing only a shrivelled head peering blearily over the top.

Matchstick legs cradle the instrument, and bird-like claws skitter nervously over the keys and buttons.

Quinn's head looks as if it's been recently severed and placed on top of the accordion. Like the head of some medieval martyr. Dead eyes and blank face strengthen the illusion.

Eventually, a small, tidy foot taps unevenly, the fingers move nimbly, and out of the great box come the hesitant strains of 'The Rakes of Mallow'.

The crowd of Irish men and women collected round the main bar jeer the sightless musician without pity.

I feel ill at ease.

Not sensitive they to physical imperfection, handicap or weakness in others, confirming my long-held belief that we, the Irish, despite the honeyed talk, the laughs, the jokes, the professed humanity and alleged deep love of country and family, are amongst the cruellest of races.

The Irish come to places like this for comfort: an oasis amid unforgiving Englishmen who don't understand them. They are, for the most part, rough, lumbering creatures mainly employed in the construction industry.

The women are there too: sharp-faced, beehive-headed, owning grand hips for childbearing, and are usually employed in domestic service; nursing or some other variety of white slavery.

Genetically hard-drinking, impulsive souls, the Irish gather here with others who share no love of order or discipline, in search of anything that the English appear to frown upon. This is the ancient notion of 'craic', an essential element of the Scattering.

Sometimes 'craic' translates into criminal behaviour, but whatever happens . . . happens.

Keep her lit!

Don't schlow down!

Keep 'er movin'!

Give 'er a lash!

Knock 'er down and make 'er take it.

I'm sitting beside Eddie Rush, who understands. We are friends. After a fashion.

He has, at that time, just re-established himself as a bricklayer, having spent the last four years of his life in prison for the crime of embedding a hatchet into the skull of a man of pure Jamaican blood.

This impetuous act resulted in a swift and relatively painless death, the significance of which appeared to have had little effect on Eddie's sunny disposition.

I am talking to a murderer.

I broach the subject diplomatically.

'Eddie,' I say, 'I believe you're a fuckin' murderer.'

He bites his lip and sniffs. 'Technically,' he replies.

'What do you mean, technically?' I cry. 'You killed a man with a hatchet!'

'Axe,' he corrects. 'Well, I suppose I did. But, Jazus, I was only done for manslaughter. I didn't mean to do it.'

'You didn't mean to do it? You lifted a hatch . . . axe and buried it in a man's head by accident? What happened?'

'We wuz on a buildin' site,' he says. 'The axe was jus' lying aroun'. I wasn't responsible for me actions. I had a fierce hangover.'

'Oh, that's all right then. Perfectly understandable. You had a hangover. The judge would understand that. Probably takes a drop himself. Happens to all of us. A bit too much the night before. Wake up with a sore head. Go to work and axe a workmate to death. I'm surprised you were in court at all!'

'I got off light on a technicality,' he murmurs. 'I was lucky. Jazus, if I'd killed a white man I'd a been in real trouble!'

I think it wise to say no more.

Eddie then shows me his boots.

'See dem boots,' he says, pointing proudly downwards to what appears to be particularly sturdy footwear. 'Got them off of a dead man, too!'

'Not the man you killed, I hope.'

'No, anudder fella. Poor bastard hanged himself in the cellar of a house we wuz knocking down. We found 'im danglin' dere. He'd bin dere for about six months, by the state of 'im. Nobody would go near 'im. I offered to cut 'im down and bundle 'im away for a tenner.'

'How could you do that?' I say, genuinely horrified but not particularly surprised.

'Easy! Ya don't tink about the smell when the bits are fallin' off 'im. I couldn't resist 'is boots though. His feet came off with them but I scraped them out . . .'

He holds up a boot, lovingly.

It isn't every day I get to talk to a murderer who is proudly displaying footwear that has been ripped from the unresisting feet of a putrefying corpse.

The club itself was a fairly harsh environment.

The bouncers were especially unforgiving.

Poles, Italians and blacks were not allowed in. So much for the lessons of tolerance, equality and humanity learnt during the course of the Great Irish Diaspora.

I remember a hapless drunk being thrown roughly down the stone steps into the street. No big deal.

The drunk, not yet entirely unconscious, had raised himself on one elbow and directed a wounding remark towards the bouncer who had ejected him so forcibly from the premises. Exhausted by the utterance of these final venomous words, the drunk then collapsed, head lolling over the rim of the pavement on to the road.

The enraged bouncer jumped into his nearby car and gunned it in the direction of the hanging head, sparks flying from hubcaps as the wheels ground against the kerb.

Luckily for him, the drunk's body was pulled back in the nick of time by nervous onlookers.

Later, I mentioned the incident to the owner, indicating my disquiet at this attempted murder.

'Oh, he won't be back,' he said, dismissively.

'I'm glad to hear it,' I said. 'He nearly decapitated the poor bastard.'

'Jazus, no. Not the bouncer! He's sound as a bell. The other fella's barred. Can't hold his drink!'

Neither could I, but I didn't expect to be murdered for it.

Eventually to Canada, playing small-time bars and clubs in Northern Ontario mining towns where it was sometimes necessary to separate band from punters by means of chicken wire stretched across the front of the stage. This acted as a shield against the beer bottles and other missiles that were hurled in our direction.

Common practice, apparently. Not to be taken personally.

But all that was behind me now. I had finally made it. Sitting in the Nickelodeon in Toronto amid the fading wisps of the Hawk's cigar smoke, I knew that things would be different from now on. No more shite-house gigs and taking abuse from Cro-Magnon Man.

And things *were* different.

At a party marking an album launch I remember flitting to and fro in a haze of illegal substances, finally spotting the figure of the most famous singer/songwriter of all sitting alone in a corner wearing a skullcap and resembling a youngish Methuselah.

I sat down beside him and eagerly told him all about what was going on in Ulster, a revolution in an ersatz democratic society, what that really meant, and how somehow he should get himself involved and come with me and I'd show him a thing or two about what protest was really about; never mind all that Woody Guthrie Dustbowl crap and spoilt American middle-class kids burning their draft cards because their parents wouldn't loan them the Thunderbird on a Saturday night. Never mind all that.

Let him come with me and see some real Voortrekker oppression brutal stuff. Dysfunction in a democratic state ruled by maniacs elected lawfully by voters who were even worse. Sharpen his edge. Get him going again . . .

I waited for a reply.

None came.

On closer examination of the Master's hooded eyes, all became clear.

There was nobody home.

Shame.

The night of my debut finally arrived.

Taking the stage with the legendary Ronnie Hawkins and the Hawks would really be something.

Heart thudding, I waited whilst Ronnie gave the crowd his schtick.

Cigar in corner of mouth, stetson on head, he screamed to the crowd of attractive, young, well-nourished Canadians:

'Now, boys and girls, before we rock 'n' roll, a little treat for y'all. Come up here . . . Mama Chickey!'

From the back of the club emerged a small, fat, repellent woman in her seventies with nylons gathered about her ankles. She was wearing an old-fashioned pinafore.

As she mounted the stage and succumbed to a crushing hug from the Hawk, she smiled to reveal a vast toothless mouth.

The Hawk shrilled, 'Maaaaaa-maaaaa Chickey from Noo Orle-ans! The last of the Red-Hot Mommas! Git downnnn!'

He handed her the microphone and bounded nimbly off-stage.

She looked directly at me, rolled her eyes and extended the longest tongue I had ever seen in my life . . . the tongue of an anteater.

Thrusting her pelvis forward obscenely, she began to sing; 'DROPKICK ME JESUS THROUGH THE GOAL-POSTS OF LIFE.'

The band and I straggled in and tried to follow the rasping vocal as she made her slovenly way across the stage, bumping and grinding to the beat, shaking what remained of her breasts.

I hadn't expected this.

Out of the corner of my eye, I saw, at the back of the unruly crowd, the upper body of a bouncer struggling with something below his waistline.

He seemed to be manhandling what could only be a large, dangerous dog towards the exit.

When he reached a break in the crowd, I saw that he was ejecting a vigorously protesting dwarf whose feet were literally not touching the ground. As he urged the screaming dwarf down the stairs, he passed a figure that looked horribly familiar to me.

It was a man wearing a close-fitting black matelot's outer

garment and an unmistakable little round hat with tassles, adorned with familiar symbols.

It was a Portuguese sailor puking on the stairs.

I waited for the flash of a knife.

This is where I came in.

Maybe it was time to think about finding a new occupation.

BROTHERS AND
OTHERS

TROUBLE WAS, I hadn't been educated for much else. Due to an early error of judgement on my part, I had found myself, at the age of twelve, in the gnarled hands of the Irish Christian Brothers. I had only myself to blame.

My two older brothers had gone to grammar school but were forced to curtail their studies as a result of separate accidents. One lost an eye courtesy of a stray shard of rock thrown up by a roadside pneumatic drill, whilst the other had recurring problems following a kick to the head sustained during a school football match.

I therefore associated grammar school with physical pain, uncertainty, anguish and the cruelly unexpected.

I was determined to have none of it, but found myself in the unfortunate position of having passed the eleven-plus examination with, as they say, 'flying colours'.

This was a great blow, and presented me with seemingly unsurmountable problems. Furtive enquiries amongst my peers led me to the conclusion that no one in the history of education had ever before been disappointed by success in the eleven-plus and, furthermore, no one could conceive of the possibility that a working-class child would refuse to go to grammar school on the grounds that the child thought he would end up in hospital because of it.

Who could I turn to?

Not to my parents, to whom the slim chance of an advanced

education was an unimaginable prize. They were good, innocent, decent people, not at all disappointed at my older siblings' failure to clear all the hurdles. They were too human for that and were contented, relieved and genuinely thankful that my two brothers had recovered and were intact. Bugger grammar school.

I, as the youngest and last boy child, was their final hope. My mother particularly was keen on my becoming a 'scholar'. She wasn't quite sure how the system operated but instinctively knew that it was better than the one she had endured.

In 1920, practically illiterate and sixteen years old, she had walked barefoot for fifteen miles from a barren farm in Donegal to the old hiring-fair in Stroke City (called the Rabble), where she stood shivering and alone on the grimy cobblestones amid the brazen cries of competing trick-o'-the-loop men, cant-men (brash con-men whose descendants are now fronting TV game shows), strong-men, tinkers, gypsies, rogues and tricksters. A jaunty farmer, sporting a shiny bowler hat and gold watch-chain, selected her from a line of other serfs, felt her arm muscles, examined her teeth, and told her to hop on to the back of his horse-drawn cart with her little bundle of personal possessions clutched tightly to her chest.

When he'd finished in the pub, he mounted the cart, gave the nag a drunken lash and trundled off into the night to his dairy farm in Co. Antrim where my mother worked a full uninterrupted six months for the total sum of £4 plus bed and board.

She laboured daily from six o'clock in the morning until eight o'clock at night and wasn't allowed to sit at any stage, even during silent meal-times.

Sometimes she and the other girls were allowed to go for a short walk on Sundays.

This was her way of life for years until she moved to Stroke City to work in shirt factories that were little more than sweat-shops. Conditions were marginally better there and sometimes the married women even got a day or two off to give birth to their children.

She sensed there must be another way, and education seemed the only forward option. How could I refuse to go to grammar school, especially after the effort that had gone into getting me this far?

I had been taken ill six months before the eleven-plus and was confined to bed by a mystery illness which was described as a 'physical breakdown'.

I first became aware that something was wrong during a talk on religion given at primary school by a spectacularly bald priest who had a very red head. He was cheerfully describing the Fires of Hell, as I remember, and making a pretty respectable stab at outlining the range of excruciating pain we could eventually expect to endure from the flames of that great institution.

He used the old Christmas Tree Analogy.

I had heard this one before. It was quite popular amongst the more imaginative members of the clergy.

Knowing our ignorance of temperature extremes measured in Fahrenheit or Centigrade, he chose to describe the excessive degree of hellish heat due to be posthumously applied to our naked, yielding flesh as 'hotter than that of a thousand burning Christmas trees'. Neat touch that. Yuletide pleasure converted seamlessly into unimaginable pain . . . the Roman Catholic way.

He proceeded gracefully from 'Scorching' to 'Humiliation by Scourging', and seemed pleased that many of us looked frightened. After all, that was why he was there.

Winding up, he fired questions concerning dogma at us. He finally got around to pointing a finger my way and, as trained, I obediently stood up.

As I got to my feet, I felt odd and barely heard the question that he spat from his lips. Something about the wraith-like nature of the Holy Ghost, as I recall.

He repeated the question.

This time his voice sounded like a faint bat-squeak in the

distance as a quickening roar filled my ears, the world tilted alarmingly sideways, then turned completely upside down, and there was I lying crookedly on the dusty floor, aware, but unable to move. I had, as they say, taken a turn, but did not, as is usually the case, show signs of a quick recovery.

He drove my inert but dully functioning body home in his priestly Hillman Minx and the doctor was called.

I was declared deathly ill, and after a short spell in hospital was allowed home on condition that I stayed in bed for what seemed a very long time indeed. Absolute rest was the apparent recipe for the restoration of rude health.

My mother was distraught, but I felt fine, except that every time I tried to sneak out of bed my spindly legs gave way under the groaning weight of my six-stone body.

I finally accepted my horizontal predicament, set to the task of reading all my father's dusty old books to pass the time, and never did discover the nature of my illness.

People didn't tell children things in those days, and even now when I ask my mother what was wrong with me when I was a kid (she's ninety-five and still angry) she says she doesn't remember exactly. Something with a 'medical name'.

This gruelling bout with a 'medical name' did not hinder my education. A kindly teacher saw to it that my lessons continued whilst I remained supine. He called two afternoons a week and set me lengthy, complicated, academic tasks that would prepare me for the eleven-plus. This occupied and improved what little there was of my mind.

When examination time loomed, my mother sought the advice of our family doctor about the advisability of my rising Lazarus-like to appear at the examination hall.

He was a nasty, patronising bastard who wore plus-fours and normally talked to us as if we were something he had just scraped off the sole of his shoe.

His surgery had a dreary Dickensian darkness about it and he maintained a flea-ridden dog that was fond of sleeping on the rug draped over the examination couch. When the doc asked patients to climb up on to the couch for medical inspection, they had to shoo the dog off themselves. I called him Dr Mengele. Our family hated him but we had to use him.

People didn't complain in those days.

Dr Mengele, displaying his usual lack of tact, informed my mother that I should not attempt to sit the eleven-plus as there was no point in 'flogging a dead ass'.

From that moment on, my mother, enraged by the good doctor's choice of words, was determined that I would appear at the examination hall. The ass would rise, flog-free.

And so it came to pass that I tottered into the designated great hall and completed the papers in half the time it took the others. They had wasted valuable months being distracted by playing football, climbing trees, kissing girls, raiding orchards, picking gooseberries, swapping conkers and shouting rude things at crippled pensioners.

I had no such distractions. I was a professional ... a damaged font of knowledge.

The others didn't have a chance.

And now, eventually fit again, I didn't want to go to grammar school.

I had been sick long enough. Why take a further risk?

The Irish Christian Brothers are a religious order formed, when the world was young and uncomplicated, for the purpose of educating the children of the poor, the confused and the halt.

Unfortunately, in the late fifties children weren't as poor and miserable as they should have been, but there were still enough of them malingering about the streets to make the Brothers' efforts worth the trouble.

I independently decided to visit them in their lair. I couldn't think of an alternative.

The Order operated what was then known as a 'technical school' for would-be future artisans who theoretically weren't up to the intellectual rigours of grammar school. I would hide there and do woodwork. That was the plan.

I had always thought of them as failed priests, and they

certainly had a sadness and a detached manner about them that led the average white boy to speculate that they would have preferred either to have died, or, alternatively, hurled for Ireland, rather than teach spotty and often smelly children. Their eyes often brightened when they spoke of Gaelic games and the prospect of a United Ireland.

They also had the reputation of being vicious bastards.

All this was far from my mind as I beat a lone path to their door. Consulting no one, I had decided to ask them to take me in as a pupil.

If they didn't want me I'd have to go to grammar school, the reportedly hideous St Columb's College, run by real priests whose alleged dark mission was to herd pliant young boys towards the priesthood ... like lemmings to the precipice.

Those who did not have it in them to become priests were made teachers or, as a last resort, poets and politicians.

All I had to look forward to there was serious physical injury and no woodwork.

I am astonished now at these early signs of undeflectable determination, iron will and bloody single-mindedness. It was the last time I was ever so. I was reeling towards a disaster of my own making.

The Brothers' living quarters were adjacent to the school, which was situated high on a hill overlooking the meaner, greyer streets of Stroke City, and I felt my heart thump as I feebly rapped on the great wooden front door with a tiny clenched fist.

A frightened-looking girl opened the door, and when I asked to see a Brother she immediately told me to go away, looking furtively behind her in the direction of the innards of the house.

A voice boomed from inside.

'Who is it, Bridget?' Bridget was obviously one of the Brothers' skivvies.

'It's a little fella!' the skivvy answered, making fluttering movements with her hands, waving me away. Like I was a moth.

'Let's have a look at him,' came the voice, and the sound of it drew nearer.

A bulky man filled the doorway, white shining collar standing out in relief from attire that was black from neck to toe. A small, improbable dog padded in his wake. The skivvy had retreated . . . walking backwards.

A Big Brother, he was three times my size and glared down at me through fierce blue eyes, feet planted firmly apart as he absent-mindedly slid his thumbs around within the confines of a black cummerbund.

'You're not one of ours!' he roared, and looked down at me more intently over the top of his little round glasses. 'Are you?'

'No,' I stuttered.

'So, what can we do for you, lad? Make it quick.'

He quickly whipped off his little round glasses, grabbed a fistful of chalkdust-coated cassock from the region of his knee and rubbed the lenses with some violence.

I noticed he smelled of tobacco.

My mouth opened and closed soundlessly . . . a guppy.

'Speak, lad! Heaven knows, God made the days short enough!'

I found the wind. My faint voice piped approximately the following: 'I want to go to your school because I don't want to end up in hospital with me leg in plaster and a broken arm or a lump out of me head or laid up sick for months because I had enough of that and I know what it's like and me mammy knows nothing about it and she doesn't even know I'm here 'cos she wants me to go to St Columb's College 'cos I passed the eleven-plus and everything and out of a sick bed as well into the bargain but it's all right for her 'cos she doesn't have to do it and you do do woodwork don't you 'cos they don't do that in the college . . . don't they not?'

I stopped, bit my lip, and probably visibly withered as he leaned down towards me, rubbing his chin.

I remember noticing something strange about his eyes as he

stared into mine from close range. They revealed a twinkle, but not just an ordinary twinkle. It was a twinkle tinged with madness. I was to see this again . . . often.

'Get a holt of yourself,' he whispered softly. 'You've passed the eleven-plus, you say?'

My adrenalin kicked in again. 'Yes, but I don't want to go to the college 'cos I want to go to your school instead. Is that all right?'

He wrapped a brawny arm lightly round my shoulders. 'You're like a wee fella who would require a bit of a glass of lemonade and some class of a biscuit, aren't you, boy, eh?'

I supposed I was.

He led me down the hallway and sharp left into a wooden-floored room that smelled lightly of paraffin oil and bacon. It was austerely furnished. Just a dark oval table and six or seven stiff-backed leather armchairs perched upon a linoleum-coated floor.

No living quarters these, I thought . . . this was an interrogation room.

I had read *The Scourge of the Swastika* and *Knights of the Bushido* when I was sick and I didn't like the look of this. There were ominous cabinets, chests of drawers, presses, and tall glass-fronted bookcases lining the walls. My imagination overheated at the thought of what they might contain . . . arcane incunabula containing methods of determining whether heretics were lying or otherwise, tests of faith, practices employed during the Spanish Inquisition, sketches of thumbscrews, branding irons . . .

Get a holt of yourself, he had said.

I did.

'Take a seat!' he commanded, and left the room.

Feet clumped down the hall, followed by the squeak of a door opening and some faint mutterings.

I waited, idly swinging my legs, acutely aware that the leather on the seat adhered sickeningly to the bare flesh exposed by the riding up of my short trousers.

Big Brother returned.

He was not alone . . . other Brothers accompanied him.

There were five or six of them, identical in their eerie cassocks. They seemed to float rather than walk. An aroma accompanied them. Of carbolic soap.

They filed in politely in an almost military manner, did not acknowledge my presence, and quietly settled on the remaining seating.

There was an awkward silence.

They studied me with obvious curiosity . . . like crows surrounding the discarded shining silver cap of a milk bottle.

On mature reflection, it's obvious what had transpired. Imagine Big Brother, having planted me safely in the front dungeon, rushing into whatever adjoining den his fellow Brothers habitually occupied.

Imagine the exchange.

'Hey, lads! COME QUICK! I've got a live one in here . . . little fella . . . completely insane . . . babbling about not wanting to go to the college . . . wants to be taught by us . . . out of his box . . . on his own too! . . . it's his idea! . . . parents don't know he's here at all . . . obsessed by WOODWORK! . . . not a word of a lie . . . would I make this up? . . . have a look at 'im . . . but go easy, don't scare him or he might bolt! . . . Follow me, come on! Quick, lads! . . . '

When they had all settled, the defeated skivvy crept in bent almost double and handed me a glass of lemonade and a fig roll.

Like a magician, Big Brother pulled out a packet of Senior Service untipped cigarettes from some concealed pocket on his person, extracted a fag, lit up with a match taken from a large box bearing the Swan legend, took a deep drag, picked a troublesome bit of tobacco from his lip, and wiped it off on his faded cummerbund.

He threw back his head with an exaggerated jerk, and exhaled noisily, directing a stream of acrid smoke towards the lime-coloured ceiling. 'So,' he said. 'What's your name, child?'

It began.

They got it all out of me.

I emptied my soul to them ... everything: fears, doubts, aspirations, dread of unavoidable grammar-school physical disfigurement, love of woodwork ... the lot.

After an hour or so, I was patted on the head and told to go home.

Wheels obviously turned behind the scenes, and although my parents were surely told of my solo mission, no mention was ever made of it to me. Come summer's end my parents informed me, a little too casually, that I was going to the Christian Brothers' technical school.

Served me right for dabbling in matters about which I knew nothing.

My first impression of the Irish Christian Brothers was that their main aim in educational life was to break the spirit of the more unorthodox and free-thinking city boys ... the sheep would cluster together and look after themselves.

Not that I regarded myself as one of the former ... I just, well, noticed the tendency.

Means used to break the spirit were varied.

Sport was a major tool. Pale, spindly-legged boys from Stroke City, accustomed only to back-street soccer and gable-end cricket, were herded on to alien green pitches and there forced to play traditional Irish ball-games with which they had little familiarity.

The Brothers favoured the big country lads who came to the school from outlying districts, and marshalled them to play against the city boys with the clear objective of damaging as many of us as possible.

This experience would 'make men' out of us. We were forced to play Gaelic football and hurling.

Gaelic football is not so much a sport as a licence to kill. Consequently, we city-slickers lived in terror of the ball coming anywhere near us as it was inevitably followed by a ruck of massive-thighed, red-faced agricultural bastards who had been encouraged by those in authority to do what they themselves desperately wanted to do anyway, i.e., render us unconscious. People can be intermittently seen playing this game on Channel 4. I still cannot bear to watch it.

Hurling is worse, in that the players are actually issued lethal weapons, in the form of razor-edged, curved wooden sticks. The secondary purpose of these hurling sticks is to strike a small, hard ball towards a given destination or goal . . . the primary purpose being to decapitate or slice open the leg of the skinniest person who happens to be nearest the previously mentioned small, hard ball.

Games were usually refereed by a snarling Brother with a name like Brother Constantine Aloysius who would invariably interpret common sense as a form of weakness.

Someone like me who would sensibly avoid all contact with any kind of ball would, for my faint-heartedness, receive lacerating swipes from a reinforced leather strap wielded by the impartial referee.

Capital offences included heading the ball or dribbling with it (in other words, what came naturally to us); any suspicion of effeminacy; the lack of an urge to get even physically; any sign of consideration or mercy; and, finally, any show of disrespect towards the referee.

On a broader canvas, other methods of alienation were employed.

We were strongly encouraged to learn the Irish language.

Now, don't get me wrong, knowledge of the Irish language would be a wonderful thing if other people spoke it too, but otherwise it seemed pretty pointless to us.

We were also instilled with an Irish Republican political ethos. This took many forms. Best to provide just one example.

During the Hungarian uprising of 1956, I remember a 'religious knowledge' class given by a Brother Finnegan, a particularly virulent little man with rat's teeth and hair that bristled as if it had been transplanted from a shoe-brush. He would perch himself upon a desk, gravely gather in the skirts of his cassock, and call for a respectful silence.

Then came the lesson for the day.

'I'm supposing you've seen newsreels in the cinema about what's going on in Budapesht and I suppose you've seen the Russian tanks in the streets of Budapesht, trundling over and crushing the bodies of the fallen fighters of the Resistance, and I suppose you're tinkin' to yourselves that that's a terrible ting altogether in itself, and I suppose you're also tinkin' how terrible it must be out in them foreign countries like Hungary where animals like the Rushkies are allowed to drive their tanks over living human beings, and I suppose you tink that that's a terrible ting too. And you'd be right.

'But mark my words, and remember this, it won't be too long before there'll be tanks like those here in your own town, and the people they'll be trundling over will be your own brothers, sisters and other loved ones.

'But mark this, and mark it well. The tanks won't be Russian, they'll be British tanks sent by Her Majesty the Queen to sort us out once and for all! And we won't stand for THAT, will we, lads?'

There was indeed a silence from the class . . . but there was a glint in the eyes of one or two of the boys, some of whom in later life were rewarded for their subsequent patriotic endeavours by very long jail terms.

I, however, survived this part of my education with very little psychological damage that I am aware of. Mainly because I didn't hear this kind of crap in the streets or at home. Only in seats of learning.

Many, though, were marked for life.

I have a mental composite image of an imaginary though not untypical boy who would, through no fault of his own, take too much of this indoctrination on board.

He will leave school to face the world armed with the following.

He will have the ability to sing 'A Nation Once Again' in D major and know the exact geographical location of all the world's needy black babies.

Conversant with the contents of the Sistine Chapel in the

Vatican Palace, he will also know how to loosely construct a wobbly wooden bedside table using only dove-tail joints.

Apart from a reluctance to eat in good restaurants because of an irrational fear that the black-suited waiter will give him a sudden clip about the ear, he will find himself occasionally, and for no good reason, uttering unconnected, grammatically suspect, snatches of the Irish language.

He will leave school with the certain knowledge that he is too short ever to play basketball professionally, will forever duck instinctively whenever he hears his name called aloud, will know exactly how to inflict excruciating pain upon small boys using a minimum of effort, and will spend the rest of his days secure in the knowledge that soccer is a game played only by occupying armies and the ideologically unsound.

Thus equipped, he will enter the adult world, eyes shining with anticipation, clutching worthless certificates with credits in Irish Language, Woodwork and Casual Labouring.

As a result of an early fixed mindset, he will never change his hairstyle and forever give the impression that his mother has just cut his hair.

He will adopt a dignified, pompous walk and disapprove of most things.

He will find himself temporarily unemployed immediately upon leaving school and use the time wisely, learning the skills necessary to become convincingly unemployed on a long-term basis.

He will blame Protestant businessmen for his failure to secure a job (usually with some justification), and learn to spit accurately on to the pavement whilst lighting a dog-end in high wind without singeing lips or fingers.

He will then master the art of playing passable snooker whilst still wetly clamping a similar dog-end between his lips.

A hump will appear on his back and he will develop bad posture.

When he is close to the terminal stage he may develop an interest in horse-racing, pigeon breeding or the training of greyhounds.

Because he has nothing else to do he may throw stones or worse at the British Army and Orangemen.
This will be deemed innocent good fun.
Someone he doesn't know may eventually hand him a gun.

FACTS ABOUT FAIRIES

NONETHELESS, ALL THINGS considered, the people of Northern Ireland have access to the best education system in the British Isles and use it skilfully to turn out maniacs and a disproportionate number of dazed zealots.

No wonder the place is a mess.

All times are troubled times in Northern Ireland.

Nothing lets up and the brink is always near.

Troubled times become more troublesome because of the various nervous ceasefires, which intermittently compel people to make a stab at behaving like rational human beings for a change. It isn't always easy, of course . . . sometimes the tourists are watching.

Ceasefires are difficult because there are certain things the natives can't forget. In a poisoned society like ours there are strange sights to be seen and heard that don't leave the mind easily.

Where else would senior representatives of the political wing of a terrorist group call for a ban on teenagers playing with air pistols because they frighten the old people, yet turn a blind eye when their own people blow away an armoured car plus passengers, courtesy of a shoulder-mounted rocket launcher used in a busy city-centre street bustling with shoppers and their children?

Or, as was the case in the small market town of Omagh, Co. Tyrone, just blow away everybody in the immediate vicinity?

Or where else would you see, at the vanguard of murderous mobs of drunken, crop-headed thugs, elegantly tailored elected politicians warning the forces of law and order of the consequences if the beasts lurch out of control, when it is the elegantly tailored elected politicians themselves who are responsible for mobilising and organising these same scumbags in the first place?

Imagine the leader of the Conservative Party in Britain urging a snarling ruck of skinheads up Downing Street and letting them loose. This is what we have to deal with here . . . the antithesis of democracy. The good people shrug their shoulders . . . powerless. There are too many of the other kind . . . on both sides.

A ceasefire is difficult in front of such a backdrop.

Nerves become frayed.

Some people can't forget the reality, which is that, for no particularly good reason, a significant proportion of the population hate the guts of another equally significant proportion of the same population, and both are prepared to do something evil and final about it.

Sensible middle-of-the-road political parties wither and die, newly minted university graduates flee the country at the first opportunity, politicians scurry like plague rats, engaged in the never-ending task of concealing the unpalatable truth, and grim-faced local television reporters stare doggedly from our screens, frightening the meek with those curious doom-laden cadences as they endlessly analyse and second-guess the sly words of those same jumped-up, opportunistic, wannabe politicians who, if it weren't for the 'Troubles', would still be playing crooked snooker in rusting, dank, corrugated-iron huts or hustling pound coins in back-street card schools under the constant, weary surveillance of a normal peace-time police force that would swiftly recognise them as the wideboys they undoubtedly are.

The future is uncertain, nobody tells the truth, and the world foolishly offers advice.

*

All this appears remote from where I sit, which is in a corner of a small, rough-hewn, one-roomed eighteenth century country cottage in West Donegal under the shadow of a major mountain that can only be described as magical. The silence drifts in from outside and only the crackle of twigs upon the open peat fire breaks the glorious quiet.

The cottage shows no sign of twentieth-century influence, and as I sit in an indoor twilight, bereft of the benefit of electric light, I nurse in my grateful hand a small, odd-shaped glass filled with a lethal substance known as poitín, i.e., illegally manufactured local whiskey of the most clear and potent kind ... too much of which can render a man permanently blind and temporarily insane.

It is straight, high-proof alcohol untroubled by a mixer. I have been drinking it for some time now on this fine, clear day.

The liquid is literally witch's brew, given to me by a rotund, smooth-complexioned lady of indeterminate age who maintains a great mane of red hair tied loosely, in a bun, to the back of her skull.

She tells me she is a white witch who specialises in the welfare of fairies.

She has no reason to lie to me. I am no tourist. I am practically a local. She knows I'll entertain no leprechaun crap. I have been round the block a number of times and she is well aware of this.

I therefore have good reason to believe that she believes what she says.

By her manner she makes it clear that she doesn't care whether I believe her or not.

I think I do believe her ... in a way.

The setting seems right. It's an Irish *Brigadoon*.

Outside the front door a brook babbles (really) and threads its way through twisted scrub that is untended by human hand. The terrain is uneven; dotted with small, sheep-infested hillocks, odd-shaped rocks and bulbous trees with stark, dead, extended claws for branches.

A heavy mist drifts slowly down from the major mountain. A donkey ambles by trailing a large erection.

The white witch asks me how things are in the north (which actually is geographically south of our present location) and as I have no desire to engage in dialogue about Contentious Orange Feeder Parades, children being burned to death in their beds, the doctrine of Parity of Esteem, parallel decommissioning of weapons, dole-signing dead-eyed tattooed patriots, screaming harridans, British Army brutality, or the very real possibility of enthusiastic ethnic cleansing taking a hold before the turn of the millennium, I sigh, and mumble that it could be worse; which indeed it always can be and usually is.

She is extremely intelligent, wears a loose-fitting gingham dress and tells me that in a previous life she was the right-hand woman of a well-known Eastern potentate until opulence bored her . . . though the last proper job she had was helping to hunt rogue members of a cocaine cartel in the jungles of Colombia . . . no dreamy-eyed sixties casualty she.

A low appreciative whistle escapes my pursed lips, but she ignores it and gazes distractedly at a small, smoke-stained window.

What a woman, I muse.

No Tupperware parties for this baby.

As the level of poitín in my glass gradually falls yet again, we talk more seriously about her fairies.

We, so to speak, delve into elves.

She discourses with the quiet authority of a university don and tells me of her direct connection to the little people, revealing that they come to her because she and the environmental conditions are considered favourable.

Fairies apparently like small, twisted trees, shrubbery for cover, running water, and rocks to clamber over. All these and more are on her doorstep, of course. They just love the locale . . . a kind of fairy Benidorm.

She claims that they like and trust her because the vibrations are right.

She plunges into detail concerning fairy physiognomy. There are three varieties of fairy extant, she reveals.

Some are small, quiet, and given to wearing interesting clothing which she describes as resembling monk's cowls. These small, hooded entities prefer to keep very much to themselves and make little or no sound as they wander around . . . barefoot, by all reports. I venture that they would make excellent neighbours.

She concurs.

Another variety of fairy is chirpy and troublesome, sounding more like the traditional elf by virtue of its preferred headgear, which she discloses as being a small pointed hat. I am somewhat thrown by the subsequent revelation that this brand of fairy is given to wearing anoraks, prompting an immediate enquiry as to where she supposed a fairy would find itself a new anorak.

She smiles lazily, re-filling my now empty glass with more firewater.

I nod limply in thanks.

I am then told about the Big Fairies. They don't come around much any more, she says, but are due sometime in the near future. Big Fairies are approximately fifteen feet tall, have pleasant faces, and are uniformly dressed in what used to be called 'long-johns', a type of body suit of underwear that comes complete with trap-door at the back for obvious purposes.

I suggest it might be difficult for a fifteen-foot fairy to make his way about the countryside undetected and that I could foresee a set of circumstances whereby I suspected the giant little person might be noticed by casual passers-by.

She replies that they are careful when travelling and take certain precautions on which she refuses to elaborate.

She also tells me that Big Fairies have very bad tempers. I postulate that this could be a dangerous trait in a fifteen-foot fairy.

After some thought, she agrees.

At this point, darkness is almost upon us, my head spins as

a result of too much poitín, and my eyes are drifting in and out of focus.

She piles on the detail.

Fairies do not speak English, of course. They converse only in Irish and have a strong aversion to electricity, heavy-metal music and people who smoke.

Fumbling for my own cigarettes, I reflect that I once had a landlady like that in Dublin.

For reasons best known to herself, she then breaks into what sounds to me like some kind of bastardised Gregorian chant . . . a form of low semi-musical wail that is both beautiful and blood-curdling.

My reaction to this is to tumble heavily from my chair on to the earthen floor, but I manage to scramble upright in time to follow her as she drifts gracefully in the direction of the doorway.

Once outside, I notice that we are being watched by the donkey I spotted earlier. Its eyes shine like fire in the moonlight and I am relieved to observe that its erection has receded. The donkey's name is Finbar.

The keening ceases abruptly. Her head jerks suddenly to the left. The donkey's head swivels simultaneously. This dual awareness of something I cannot detect unnerves me.

'They're here!' she whispers urgently.

'Not the fifteen-footers!' I cry.

'No, the others,' she rasps. 'They want to see you.'

I scan the immediate vicinity. Not an anorak in sight.

'Can they see me from here?' I enquire.

'No, the conditions do not prevail,' she answers.

'Well, can't you p...p...pervail 'em?' I slur. My condition is worsening at an alarming rate.

'Yes,' she says quickly. 'Sit on this.'

She plonks me down on a three-legged wooden milking stool and runs indoors, reappearing moments later with a strange-shaped bottle from which she sprinkles a white powder, forming a circle that encloses my rapidly deteriorating form.

'They'll see you now!' she declares triumphantly.

I sit quietly on my perch, remaining upright with a fair degree of difficulty. Nothing happens.

'Nothing's happening,' I say.

'Be patient. They're watching you,' mutters my witch slowly. 'Don't do anything that might alarm them.' She points at an ugly clump of moss-covered rocks and nods sagely.

I sit still, staring at the blurred boulders for what appears to be a very long time, and then must have fallen asleep. The next thing I recall is coming to slumped in a wicker armchair inside the cottage.

'Wha' happened?' I enquire thickly.

She sits beside the fire, gently disturbing the embers with an iron poker of some antiquity.

She turns to me and smiles.

'They liked you,' she says, with some satisfaction. 'They told me so.'

'But I didn't see them,' I whine.

She leans back and stretches slowly, like a cat.

'It's your own fault, isn't it?' she says slowly. 'You will insist on smoking.'

A close encounter with non-smoking fairies. Why don't the little fuckers emigrate to America like all the other decent Irish people? Non-smokers are appreciated there.

Donegal is like that.

It's a paradise for those who hear a different drummer . . . a sensible place where anything goes; a world away from hate-torn, intolerant, mad Ulster next door.

Donegal is Europe's best-kept secret, though Americans have long known about it and there are worrying signs that the word has spread to Japan. But that's OK.

There's room for everybody.

It's where people go when the world moves too rapidly for their liking.

Need a white witch? Require the services of a druid? Want to contact a carver of didgeridoos, a tree-worshipper, a bulk patchouli oil dealer, a thong manufacturer, a bogus osteopath, a healing seventh son of a seventh son, a clutch of stranded gentry? Fancy half a pig's head (shaven or unshaven, sir?), a gallon of buttermilk, a fistful of dope, a second-hand hookah? Look no further.

I've had long experience of this locale, having spent many childhood summers with my two silent, elderly bachelor uncles in a small, decrepit family farmhouse that still clings stubbornly to a barren East Donegal hillside where it has nestled relatively unchanged for nigh on four hundred years.

My uncles felt no need to communicate verbally with each other and disappeared daily mid-morning into separate fields, allegedly to perform vaguely agricultural tasks. I was left alone and gloriously happy during the rest of the day . . . just me, my friends the free-range chickens, dog Gyp, and a horse called Bob.

My uncles and I got together for evening meals . . . stiff, awkward affairs, punctuated only by the ticking of an antediluvian clock and the audible munching of badly decayed teeth upon jacketed, boiled potatoes which were carefully selected from a pile of steaming tubers heaped in the middle of a knotted wooden table otherwise bare, except for a small mound of loose salt and a sturdy jug of the thickest buttermilk.

Masticating slowly, flat caps delicately balanced on the edges of stout knees, they existed in a twilight zone that even I, at this tender age, sensed as something awesome and timeless . . . a living history lesson in that, down the centuries, this was more or less the way things had always been.

Primitive, quiet and dull.

This was the way things must have been before the Great Famine, just before there was an America to go to, where good men from this parish could kill Indians for sport and get medals for their trouble.

My uncles told me tales of the Famine, as if it had happened yesterday, which in a sense it had; their granny (my great-grandmother) had survived it and talked to them about little else when they were children . . . that's close.

My uncles weren't used to children and I was treated like a small, deformed adult.

They felt a genetic need for strong drink every Saturday night and often took me with them . . . to Buncrana, a small fishing town no more than six miles distant.

The three bicycles would set off in formation down a leafy, rutted lane in the direction of the main artery, which was only slightly less leafy and rutted.

No words were exchanged as rusty wheels were forced complainingly through occasional layers of unyielding gravel. I normally lagged behind after a while, spindly legs pumping hard in a bid to avoid dropping even further back before mercifully the lights of the settlement loomed.

Brakes eventually squealed and bicycles were propped against the gable wall of Bradley's Public House and Victuallers or, alternatively, thrown carelessly against the railings outside Flanagan's Religious and Fancy Goods shop.

At this juncture, a silver sixpence usually flew through the air in my direction, the entrance fee to the small cinema located at the far end of the street.

Bradley's pub was situated centrally and men from outlying hills accumulated there in force, spilling out on to the street. My taciturn uncles mingled easily with them and became almost normal sociable human beings, muttering greetings to men who looked exactly like them; men wearing ill-fitting black suits shiny from wear, with obscenely broad trouser-bottoms that betrayed the ravages of a thousand rough encounters with metal bicycle clips.

It was not unusual to see fly-buttons left carelessly undone, and no outfit was complete without the mandatory grimy grey jumper, heavily flecked with cigarette ash . . . non-smokers hadn't been invented yet.

Peeking out from the tops of these jumpers jutted evidence that the upper bodies were additionally swathed in soiled, collarless grandad shirts. From the other end of the body poked black, laced-up, heavy boots displaying signs of serious abuse. Nestling within, vulnerable feet were protected from a harsh world by the thickest of dark, woolly socks.

No man was bare-headed; craniums were topped by flat-caps. Each man's cap was a window to his soul, a testament to his individuality, and the angle at which it was worn was a clue to his mood, state of mind or general philosophy of life.

I knew about angular headgear. I could read hats. I understood their language . . . I was the Hat Whisperer.

I had learnt this arcane art from my late father's homburg. He was a serious poker player and, of an evening, spotting him on his way home, I could tell by the angle of his hat not only whether or not he had been playing cards, but also whether he had won or lost.

I shared this gift with my mother who had figured it out independently.

'Where's Daddy tonight?' I would enquire.

'Where do you think?!' would be the reply. 'Not to worry,' my mother would add. 'If he wins he'll come sailing in here whistling, with the hat on the back of his head hanging on two hairs.'

And so it often was.

THE READING OF HATS . . . ELEMENTARY PRINCIPLES

1 Hat precariously on back of head, tilted upwards at impossible angle = pecuniary gain through game of chance.
2 Hat pulled forward, shadowing eyes = loss of considerable sum.
3 Hat on back of head but listing heavily to port = general feeling of contentment without necessarily the advantage of pecuniary gain through game of chance.
4 Hat on front of head but pulled severely starboard = something on his mind.
5 Hat squarely in middle of head = a workmanlike determination to achieve unknown goal.

6 Hat taken off completely = sign of utter exhaustion.
7 Hat flung angrily on to floor = room evacuated by all
  personnel.

And so on . . . many permutations. This advanced phrenology
stood me in good stead for many years and kept me a jump
ahead of my father's moods. At no time was he ever aware
that his son could read his hat.

But I digress.

I would, of course, never use my silver sixpence to gain
entrance to the cinema. Waiting for most of the men to
eventually disappear into the pub, I would then climb on to a
convenient wooden bench, from which vantage point I could
peer at the drinkers inside through a partially opened
window.

I see it still. A bald, weary, cynical, red-faced man with
mutton-chop sideburns stood behind the bar and ladled out
pints of viscous stout to rough men who never, ever said
thank you.

A man with a deeply creviced face, a shock of snow-white
hair and a gnarled walking stick, sang to the cap perched
upside down on his knee. He was keening in Irish with an
almost Moorish atonality . . . he sounded like a Commanche
medicine man.

Two wizened crones engulfed in pseudo-Sicilian black
shawls maintained the best of order for the singer whilst
intermittently ramming pinches of snuff into their noses and
noisily, forcefully snorting the stuff to its eventual destination
at the back of their brains.

A cadaverous man danced noisily, and though his upper
trunk was rigid and his arms seemingly glued to his sides,
small, dainty, nimble feet flashed like leaping salmon.
Nobody took a bit of notice.

The babble of gruff talk, the doleful singing, the stiff
dancing, the fiddle music drifting over the wooden partitions
of the snug, the thick cigarette smoke, the smell of whiskey,
porter and blazing peat, the spitting on the floor, the guttural

clearing of throats, the sudden shouts, the hyena laughter . . . all were absolutely irresistible.

And here's a thing.

Although I wasn't allowed inside, most of these people knew who I was.

They knew me as Charles's Kate's Gerald. Charles being my long-dead grandfather, and Kate my mother's name.

Considering my grandfather was born in the 1860s, that's what I call continuity.

I belonged here from way back. I was a part of this . . . and glad of it.

Round midnight I usually helped my uncles on to their bikes and followed them watchfully as they weaved home in silence, in total blackness and happiness.

Maybe the fairies were watching us.

They didn't seem to mind a drink or two.

I bade a fond farewell to the white witch and with throbbing head drove towards Northern Ireland, eventually going through the nominal border check-point manned by uninterested British soldiers who wished they weren't there, and alert, grim, pink-faced, bulletproof-vest-wearing police-men who wished the soldiers weren't there too.

Stopping to have my car refuelled by a pimply, rude youth who didn't appear to see me at all, I picked up a Belfast newspaper and my eyes fell upon a story tucked away on page 5.

It read thus:

A young man lying unconscious and critically injured on the road after a horrific car crash was stripped of his jewellery by a crowd which mistakenly believed him to be a joy-rider. He had been catapulted through the wind-screen, slamming against a brick wall.

He was relieved of his watch, bracelet and a Glasgow Celtic ring. The boy's mother was particularly upset by the fact that they even took his shoes.

The boy's father said, 'There were crowds around him. They were like vultures.'

Home, sweet home . . .

SEX AND DRUGS AND

ON THE DOLE

AND HOME, SWEET infuriating home, it will always remain. Over the last thirty years many Stroke City natives have been superficially glad to see the back of their metropolis, fleeing to settle in distant lands.

Photographs of large knots of now-prosperous Stroke City expatriates are often seen in our local newspapers; peering self-consciously at the camera, eyes squinting before a fierce foreign sun; people fatter and older than they used to be, wearing clothes that don't appear to belong to them, laughing a little too hysterically, surrounded by their foreign children; gathered round barbecues in Melbourne, Manitoba, Minneapolis, Miami or Mombasa – not entirely happy . . . the ones who got away.

But the pull remains.

I tended to avoid them in my aimless travels. Not because I didn't like them. It's more complicated than that.

I did, in atonement for past sins, attend one or two brave patriotic gatherings in remoter outposts where it was too difficult to hide, and always came away saddened.

Stroke City has marked the ex-natives in a unique way. They love their home town dearly but can't countenance the thought of living there again. They love it too much for the way things used to be. Before the scumbags made their presence felt.

To these saddened emigrant eyes, after a drink or two,

everywhere else is a mere limbo.

I, on the other hand, escaped from the city many times but always came back. I don't know why.

This time I seemed to be back for good.

It was 1975. I'd had enough of sex and drugs and rock 'n' roll on the North American continent and regarded myself lucky to have escaped with my mind more or less intact.

I'd had enough of nights lost in a haze of illegal fumes, punctuated by bouts of furious, mock-creative energy generated by the ingestion of rare chemicals, enough of bending squealing guitar strings at mind-crunching decibel levels, enough of waking up in threatening places, enough of beautiful, fucked-up, scantily clad women in search of their 'inner selves', enough of zonked-out American musicians barely able to fart without the encouragement of a noseful of cocaine, enough of consorting on a daily basis with pimps, hustlers and minor hoodlums, enough of meeting previously venerated rock 'n' roll idols only to discover feet of the crumbliest clay, enough of not requiring sleep for a straight three days, enough of travelling from city to faceless city in reckless, arrogant, hedonistic style, enough of uppers, downers, poppers, Thai-sticks soaked in opium, Bolivian Marching Powder, MDA, angel dust, crank, horse and whispered rumours about what Elvis was really like.

All in all, hugely entertaining and enjoyable, of course ... but enough was enough. It was time to take stock. The final decision was made for me by a bathroom mirror.

Heaving my aching body from a rumpled bed one rainy afternoon in an anonymous New York City hotel room after two straight days of little sleep, no food, too much thunderous music and general inspired misbehaviour, I staggered loo-wards in search of water to soothe a parched and heavily furred tongue.

Grasping the edges of the mottled sink, I happened to catch a glimpse of my reflection in the spattered glass.

The gaunt, spare outline of my face looked back at me through lifeless eyes.

I had never seen my personal skull in such stark detail before . . . normal, everyday facial flesh usually got in the way. This was no hallucination.

Rock 'n' roll was taking its toll.

Atop a haggard and skeletal body, the cadaverous skull was a chilling sight.

And it was all my own work.

This was self-inflicted emaciation on a Japanese prisoner-of-war camp scale and I didn't much care for the look of it.

This was more than just a bad hair day. It occurred to me that I was terminally fucked.

Before, I had never exactly been Mr Universe, but this degree of weight loss was serious.

My brain was sending me a warning shot across the bows.

Better heed it.

Keep this up and you die, kid.

Anyway, I was too old for this, pushing thirty and just about as far as I was going to get in this particular branch of showbusiness.

By the hideously low standards of the contemporary music industry I suppose I was doing OK, lodged near the top end of the rock totem pole, but the leap to big money and real fame was great and time was not on my side. I was merely on the edge of the shark pool.

I knew I could maintain my present position for three to four years tops, but after that lay the prospect of an inevitable slow slide down the same increasingly greasy pole to the point where I would be forced to regard my being a musician as just a job. This was fatal.

Then the nightmare would really begin: the gradual, relentless descent to the purgatory of playing in bands that existed to service bar mitzvahs, anniversary parties, Russian weddings, obscure Bulgarian rites of passage, lawyers' dress dances, plumbers' Christmas-do's, golfing rituals, and, God forbid, get-togethers for Irish expatriates.

Anyway, there is a rule of thumb in the music business which many guitar players and champions of other contemporary musical instruments choose to ignore. It goes thus:

The form of music that one has devoted one's life to mastering will immediately become unfashionable: (a) when one has finally perfected it; or (b) when one has reached one's early thirties. Furthermore, (a) and (b) are usually concurrent. Discuss.

I could see it coming. I was used to trauma, having been born at an awkward time, i.e., 1944. Experts will understand when I say that I was always an 'inbetweenie' . . . i.e., too young for Elvis and marginally too old for the Beatles. I was a misfit. Against considerable odds I had gone far. I was now on the cusp of Stage 5 in the career of an average white man dabbling in rock 'n' roll.

There are six stages in all.

STAGE ONE: *Initial Crazed Enthusiasm*

This normally begins in early teens or, in more aggressive cases, during the pre-teenage years.

The often pre-pubescent child behaves as if struck down by a rare virus. The initial infection can usually be traced to that specific defining moment in the child's life when he or she, invariably by chance, hears a particular piece of popular music for the first time. It seems to come straight from God, and few are chosen to go all the way.

Let us not confuse this phenomenon with what many civilised people may recall as their gradual introduction to, say, the works of Chopin or Beethoven; an awareness that will grow and develop over time into an appreciation of higher forms of musical achievement.

We're talking rock 'n' roll here. It's dirty and it kills. This is instant . . . wild and uncontrollable . . . visceral. The hearing of a mere snatch of this music is often enough to stun the child into submission and alter the course of his/her life forever.

It happened to me in a chip shop.

Huddled in a wooden booth with three of my pock-faced friends, sharing a solitary plate of chips, loutishly sprinkling vinegar over each other and fighting over a glass of brownish lemonade, we generally barely noticed the background wallpaper of sound that routinely emerged from the garish jukebox at the bottom of the stairs leading to the upper tier of the café, where older boys took girlfriends for the purpose of drinking watery coffee and lying shamelessly to them.

We didn't bother the jukebox much, stuffed as it was with Pat Boone crap and perennial Doris Day, Dean Martin and, worst of all, Tony Bennett. It's not that we didn't like the music, nor did we even discuss it. It just seemed that the records had been put in there for other people . . . nothing to do with us, you see.

Then I heard it.

Something so weird and wonderful that it jolted me with the force of a direct hit of lightning.

I discovered later that it was the intro to a song called 'Shakin' all Over' by Johnny Kidd and the Pirates . . . a tumbling, harsh, reckless, discordant, clashing torrent of notes played on electric guitar that immediately made the hair on the back of my head seem to shoot straight up and quiver painfully. A bout of whining singing followed the intro and then came the guitar once more . . . same hair rose again.

I disengaged myself from the lone plate of chips and beat a swift path to the jukebox where I stood, nose pressed to the Perspex, watching the tiny record revolve within the innards of the great, throbbing machine. I stared at the label and memorised both title and artist.

When the song ended, a robotic claw-arm deposited the disc back amongst the serried ranks of Boones and Bennetts.

I glanced at my friends. They seemed ready to leave and were performing the standard ritual of loosening the cap of the big glass salt bottle.

They hadn't noticed the music.

That's when I realised that something unusual had happened to me.

I had lost my soul.

For the next few weeks my sole purpose in life was the gathering of sixpences to feed the eager maw of the jukebox.

On one occasion I played 'Shakin' all Over' eighteen times in a row and was severely reprimanded by the Italian owner of the establishment. Even I had to concede that he probably had a point.

Economic sense finally prevailed when it occurred to me that, for a modest sum, I could buy the record myself and play it at home as often as I liked on the primitive family record player that fell just short of requiring an attached horn.

And so it started.

I withdrew from society and managed to talk my parents into buying me a cheap acoustic guitar with strings strung high above the fretboard, causing the tips of my fingers to blister and bleed. I didn't know the strings could be easily lowered. I didn't care. The sound was the thing.

Moving permanently into my bedroom, emerging only for hurried meals, I practised five, six sometimes seven hours a day and dreamed away the rest.

After a couple of years of this, it was time for the bird to fly.

STAGE TWO: *The Learning Curve*

It was late on a Sunday morning when the knock finally came to my door. My mother summoned me from my eyrie.

'There's a man we don't know at the door!' she yelled. And indeed there was – a nervous-looking man whose right eye twitched a little. Over his shoulder I could see, engine idling, a large, gaily painted van containing a number of men whose sleepy eyes were staring with dull curiosity in my direction.

The back end of the van was stuffed with boxes, cases, rolls of electric wire and various other unidentified metallic contrivances.

The painted legend along the side of the vehicle informed me that I was in the presence of the Imperial All-Stars

International Showband (Derry, N. Ireland).

My heart leaped.

I knew about showbands.

Rural Ireland, as a whole, was far from the hub of the entertainment industry but was slowly clawing its way into the modern age by a strange route.

Because of the almost complete absence of television in broad swathes of the country, pop music filtered in by means of the radio. Most of the pop chart acts were British or American but did not tour the perceived cultural wasteland that was the Emerald Isle.

As these original hit-generating outfits were unavailable, there was room for the Next Best Thing, which was bands of local musicians playing chart songs badly and wearing cheap suits that glittered. Primitive lounge cover bands with no lounges to play in plied their trade in huge, alcohol-free, breeze-block mausoleums hastily erected on remote, wind-blown, rural sites, i.e., dance halls . . . a uniquely Irish cottage industry.

Nevertheless, it was the only game in town.

A showband usually consisted of seven members: mad drummer, lead guitar, bass guitar, opinionated lead singer, tenor saxophone, trumpet and trombone. Thus equipped, a band could crudely ape almost any chart song.

Playing in a showband required a strong physical constitution; musical ability was secondary.

Long hours of travel over pot-holed roads left weak men racked with exhaustion. Only the strong survived to punch in five hours of spirited blowing, strumming, screaming and thumping, perched on feet-pinching white bootees with often impossibly high heels.

I had observed these men in the dole queue.

By this time, having forsaken all respectable aspirations in favour of becoming a professional guitar player, I was signing for unemployment benefit at the dole office's Casual Box 6, where my potential occupation was listed on my personal claim form as, excitingly, Routine Clerk.

I was gainfully unemployed and officially classified as a Casual Worker because I occasionally provided poor acoustic guitar accompaniment for singers in pubs, for which I was paid ten shillings a night. Not yet wise to the ways of the world, I had declared this income to the Obergruppenführer behind the dole counter, and these paltry earnings were duly deducted from my weekly stipend of four pounds and eleven shillings.

I was required to sign on at Casual Box 6 at 11 a.m. every weekday and took a keen interest in my fellow signees. The only casual work available in the economically constipated Stroke City of the time was in music and stevedoring. The long, waiting morning line was therefore made up solely of musicians and dockers ... it wasn't difficult to tell them apart.

It was a surreal queue.

The musicians, with their winkle-picker shoes, bum-freezer jackets, pencil-thin trousers, Crombie overcoats, Brylcreemed quiffs, bleary eyes, pasty complexions, hunched backs, gentle conversation and general air of ill-health contrasted strongly with the barrel-chested, mighty-limbed, weatherbeaten, oath-muttering, whiskey-sodden, fist-happy, swaggering real men who constituted the stevedoring element.

The dockers talked loudly of tonnage, rates of pay, prevailing weather conditions, the imminent arrival of spud-boats and other mighty merchantmen; whilst the musicians quietly discussed gigs, rates of pay, the musical ability of absent colleagues, the pliability of loose women encountered on the road, and how best to prolong the life of a saxophone reed.

All co-existed happily as they shuffled inexorably forwards under a dense haze of tobacco smoke.

I wanted to be one of these showband musicians, not least because many of them wore scholarly, dark-framed spectacles which I'm sure were not absolutely necessary.

And now one of them was at my door.

'You back people in the Wagon Wheel?' he barked.

He was referring to the pub in which I occasionally sheepishly appeared. I couldn't deny it.

'Yes, ' I replied tersely.

'We're stuck. Guitar player's gone down with somethin'. Can you hack the gig?'

I noticed that his hair was artfully arranged to disguise the fact that he had very little of it. Thick, greasy clumps of it had been marshalled together and hauled from a fertile region just above his right ear to cover an almost denuded pate. It was an accomplished piece of bold hair architecture.

'What do you mean?' I enquired innocently.

'Can you hack the gig?' He looked at my uncomprehending face and sighed. 'Can you play guitar with us tonight? Kiltimagh, County Mayo. Early start.'

'Oh.'

I panicked. I had never played in a real band before, never stood on a real stage, never even touched an electric guitar, never used an amplifier.

'Do you sing?' he added.

'God, no!' I replied in terror. 'Listen, I only have an acoustic guitar, I have no equipment, no amplifier, no nothing . . .'

'No problem. Use Frankie's.'

'Frankie?'

'Our guitar player. The guy that's sick.'

There was no way out. I wanted this more than anything else in the world but it was too sudden. I wasn't ready.

Or so I thought.

I was on the road . . .

This is how it usually starts.

In most case studies, what usually follows is a rough apprenticeship during which one develops the sturdy carapace that is required to persevere.

Playing when and where one can in a variety of pick-up bands of low quality, it is possible to acquire hands-on skills, but there are countless humiliations along the way.

I have played in some indescribably foul bands, one of

which consisted of four drunken accordionists, a schizo-phrenic drummer and a cross-dressing vocalist who was practically blind; in another so awful that we were pelted off-stage by a variety of coins and particularly delicious wrapped, chocolate-covered toffees; also in one doomed outfit where nightly fisticuffs between members was the norm; and in another band whose members were locked in the throes of sexual intrigue caused by three of the musicians conducting separate steamy affairs with the girl vocalist, who in turn was married to the bandleader, who in turn was understandably suspicious but constantly accused the only two men in the band who were entirely blameless. I learnt to keep my mouth firmly shut.

Nor was this an initially lucrative road to travel. Often, the bands were so bad that promoters refused to pay us. Often, when we did get paid, the bandleader wouldn't pay us; cheques bounced, heartbreaking tales of imminent financial ruin were routinely trundled out, and once, uniquely, a bandleader paid me for my night's work by presenting me with a hessian sack bulging with potatoes which he miraculously produced from the back of the van . . . King Edwards, as I recall.

None of this really mattered, of course. The main thing was that a man was learning his trade, and this can only be done on the road, in front of an audience, no matter how hostile that audience may be.

I was still living at home and consequently did not starve. That comes later.

STAGE THREE: *The Starving Years*

Being a professional musician in Stroke City meant that one did not have to sign on the dole as often as one did when one was not a professional musician.

A professional musician was one who derived the bulk of his income from the playing of music, buoyed by a small but essential weekly financial supplement gleaned from the Government by making par-for-the-course false criminal claims at Casual Box 6; one was not a professional musician if the reverse applied . . . a fine distinction, but it seemed important at the time. This practice has marked me for life to the extent that modern talk of dole fraud goes right over my head. Why not defraud a Government funded by money collected from English people? Nobody I knew paid taxes, and rightly so.

The starving began when one clinched a permanent job in a musically decent band that had been together for some time. The first inkling of the Great Hunger usually came when bands were forced to tour Irish clubs in England.

This bold move was necessitated by the onset of the annual season of Lent, when showbands fled Catholic Ireland like rats from a trap; religious tradition having decreed that all dancing must cease during that Holy Time . . . Dust Bowl time for musicians.

The season of Lent is the period of forty days lasting from Ash Wednesday to Holy Saturday, observed as a time of penance and fasting, commemorating Jesus's fasting in the wilderness.

God was obviously not a deity keen on fasting alone. Many musicians joined Him, though for different reasons. Starving during Lent was but a harbinger of what was to come . . . a useful introduction.

Six weeks of traipsing around England and Scotland (no Wales; the Irish don't like Wales . . . too much like home), financial welfare depending on the caprice of a usually demagogic bandleader who would frequently disappear for days on end with big-titted Irish nurses from Galway, was a surefire method of losing weight.

Many a carefree day was spent staring penniless through the scuffed windows of back-street Glaswegian, Mancunian or Shepherd's Bushian boarding houses, avoiding shrill, fat landladies, subsisting on a balanced diet of milk and Mars bars, waiting for news of the next gig.

Would it be a sinkhole in Camden Town, the horror that was Hammersmith on a Saturday night, or, blessed relief, the relatively plush Gresham Ballroom on London's Holloway Road with a revolving stage that left stranded drunken musicians pawing blindly in the darkness backstage as their companions sailed mechanically towards the spotlights to meet the impatient dancers out front?

We played where the emigrant Irish gathered.

Places not for the faint-hearted . . . stuffed to the rafters with navvies, misfits, tearaways and runaways who were either drunkenly, dangerously sullen or dangerously, drunkenly happy . . . all equally short-fused and inclined to chin a stranger on a whim. One learned to tread carefully in their midst.

When Irish men and women move to England, something odd occurs that causes their Irishness to alter.

The gentle, whimsical and easy-going nature that characterises most of their behaviour at home seems to disappear, and something else kicks in . . . they revert to stereotype, Old Hollywood-style.

You've seen the films . . . wooden rooms with sawdust-covered floors filled to bursting point with bearded men who shout wildly, laugh crazily or argue furiously over fuck-all.

Barry Fitzgerald tries to restrain Victor McLaglen, who has sworn to throttle John Wayne for daring to even think about defiling the honour of Maureen O'Hara.

Spencer Tracy, the local police officer, lies drunkenly asleep, sprawled over a corner table, spurned and wounded because he also wants to defile Maureen O'Hara but is too old for her to notice him at all.

The sound of music from demented fiddles fills the air . . . women in big skirts leap like gazelles as they dance in a swirling, dizzying circle, their momentum and balance controlled by wild-eyed, lust-maddened men with their sleeves rolled up.

Bottles fly, glasses crash, tankards clank, obscenities lace the air and the bartender goes about his business in the sure knowledge that eventually some unmanageable giant of a mountain-man will declare, 'No man talks to me like dat!' ... signalling the commencement of a fierce brawl in which everyone will enthusiastically take part ... a fight that will demolish the entire bar plus fixtures and fittings before spilling out on to the street.

Innocent passers-by will be flattened by great swinging fists, blood will flow freely but all will end suddenly with gory smiles displaying smashed or splintered teeth, and hearty slaps will be delivered to broad backs for, sure, wasn't it only a bit o' crack and what's life if you can't let your hair down every once in a while ... no hard feelings and balls of malt all round for the boyzzz ...

Fantasy, of course, except that in an Irish pub in Melbourne in 1990, I witnessed exactly the scene I have described above (I have used the names of veteran Hollywood stars for dramatic effect).

Things weren't as bad as that in Lenten England and Scotland, but they were close.

Six weeks isn't a long time to starve, but the experience laid solid foundations for the permanent move away from home.

During the course of one of these Lenten tours, we found ourselves playing in a vile Irish club in Manchester. The club was managed by two demolition contractors from Co. Mayo who, unaccountably, took a shine to the band, offered us a permanent job as resident 'orchestra', and promised additional opportunities to earn money if we would undertake to perform light manual work at one or other of the many ravaged buildings which they were in the process of razing to the ground.

The fact that we not only accepted this offer but actually thought it an attractive idea is a measure of how defeated, disillusioned, burnt-out and crazy we were at the time. Many character-forming experiences followed.

I learnt that it was not necessarily a good idea to wake up badly hungover in the dingy bedroom of a dilapidated house in Manchester's Moss Side to discover that I was lying beside a naked woman whose face was unfamiliar to me but who was, nevertheless, gently and patiently explaining to six furiously angry West Indians surrounding the bed that I could not possibly have jemmied and robbed the gas meter in the hallway as I hadn't been out of her sight since ten o'clock the night before and, besides, she had already searched my pockets and found them barren.

Additionally, I learnt that there is no future in light demolition work; that a man cannot make any semblance of a living by extracting six-inch nails from recycled planks on a piece-work basis; that it is extremely foolish to walk directly below Irishmen who are stripping rotting roofs; and, finally, that it is an act of suicide to work in the cellar of a building due for demolition because that is precisely when people with a highly developed sense of humour will decide to torch the place, betting largish amounts of money on how much time will elapse before the innocent cellar-worker becomes aware of the growing inferno and manages to scramble to safety . . . or not, as fate would decree.

All good, innocent fun, of course . . . the Starving and the Danger are mutually complementary.

The music part was easy.

We played four nights a week, but only for the first two or three hours of the evening; the main attraction (the touring Irish showband) took care of the final two hours.

These arrangements suited us greatly. We could experiment musically whilst the club was sparsely populated. The only patrons who turned up early were teetotallers, terminal spinsters, awkward youths just off the boat, lone lost men and the occasional odd couple who preferred an unpopulated dance floor upon which they could display, unhindered by mere mortals, an unfortunate interest in ballroom dancing.

The ballroom dancers were a pain in the arse. Since the beginning of recorded time (even before the paso doble or bossa nova), musicians have always hated ballroom dancers, not just because of those ghoulish, pasted-on smiles, but mainly because they habitually stop dead in mid-flight to stare sternly at the band if the music or tempo falls short of expectations.

We, the band, didn't give a fuck and often tried to sabotage the gliding couples by playing Bach fugues in strict waltz-time. The tempo was spot on but the unfamiliar musical content would throw them entirely, often resulting in awkward stumbles which the band would observe with some satisfaction.

Finishing early had its advantages. When the main attraction took the stage for the last two hours, we were free to stalk the club for vulnerable female prey.

By this late hour, in contrast to the other patrons, who had staggered in pissed, we were sometimes sober, smartly dressed and, by virtue of our perceived showbiz connections, desirable to women who had, as they say, a number of bottles in them. So there was much sneaking into nurses' quarters that adjoined obscure Salford hospitals; silently padding, shoes in hand, past the bedrooms of sonar-equipped landladies in Chorlton-cum-Hardy; and skilfully engineered invitations to Sunday lunch in the homes of doe-eyed English girls of Irish parentage where the welcome grub was greedily scoffed in the presence of the nervously silent paterfamilias, who was usually uneasy in the knowledge that his trusting, innocent daughter was making a major mistake.

Once in a while, though, true love struck.

Falling for a black American stripper/recreational masseuse has its obvious drawbacks, but I was blind to them at the time.

I don't know how she got past the whites-only Voortrekker door policy, but assume that her safe passage through the gorilla-infested portals was only partly due to her statuesque figure and stunning looks and probably mostly due to the fact that she was accompanied by a short, fat, ugly, cigar-smoking, dinner-suited man who looked as if he owned the place which, in this jumbled world of Irish Murphia, he almost certainly did.

It was love at first sight. She was the most exotic creature I had ever seen: tall, Afro-headed, copper-coloured and proud, hygienically wrapped in a dress of the finest clingfilm.

We were on-stage when I first saw her sail majestically by. We were having our usual nightly musicians' private snigger whilst performing a song called 'The Patriot Game'; a semi-sacred Irish Republican anthem dealing with informers, treachery and the usual unstoppable urge to be killed for one's country. The first line of the song is 'Come all ye young rebels, and list while I sing.' On the word 'list', the vocalist would angle his body at about forty-five degrees to starboard and maintain this position for the rest of the song. Childish, I know, but we enjoyed it.

A man had to be alert on stage. On one occasion, our tenor saxophonist was engrossed in a particularly intricate piece of fingerwork during the course of a jazzy solo, when he noticed his trouser leg being violently yanked by a carrot-topped man with a huge nose. 'Play "Danny Boy" for the name o' Jazus and quit that squeaky shite,' yelled Carrot-top.

Ignored completely by the sax player, the music-lover yanked more vigorously, almost loosening the proud artist's trousers from their moorings. 'Play us something fuckin' decent, in the name of Christ! Play fuckin' "Danny Boy" will ya?'

Something had to give.

I moved instinctively back out of harm's way.

The saxophonist leaned over and whispered something into Carrot-top's ear. This prompted an immediate and violent reaction which was sharply curtailed when the musician let loose a compact short right that altered the shape of the music-lover's large nose forever, propelling him a full ten yards before he collapsed in an untidy heap.

I had already removed my guitar and was planning my escape route. Rough-hewn men were making their way determinedly towards the stage. In an inspired moment, the saxophonist grabbed the microphone. 'Nobody, and I mean NOBODY, calls ME an Orange bastard! I'm a FENIAN and PROUD of it!'

I stared at him with limitless admiration.

The man was a genius.

Carrot-top was hauled away and thrown heavily down the stone steps outside.

The saxophonist beamed broadly and the drummer and I stealthily gathered up the loose change that had fallen out of Carrot-top's pockets as he had hit the deck. It's an ill wind . . .

Her name was Tina.

Eventually, I managed to corner her outside the ladies' toilet where no one would see us.

Working furiously, I managed to impress her by a combination of flattery and smooth, insincere oratory, whilst simultaneously registering the strong but false impression that I was decent, shy and quite well-off.

We arranged to meet for tepid coffee the next day.

It turned out that she liked Irish people, her father having inherited some well-documented Green Blood that coursed furiously through his otherwise perfectly acceptable Afro-Caribbean veins. Her mother was mercifully Blarney-free and just about as black as a person could be, thank you very much.

A native of Tulsa, Oklahoma, Tina told me she had been a dancer with a touring stage show and had impulsively married a stage-door Johnny in London who made himself scarce when she became heavy with child.

One thing had led to another and here she was; she could hardly believe it herself . . . stuck in sooty Manchester with a child to support.

I didn't believe a word of it, of course.

None of this mattered anyway.

What did matter was that she was a magnificent specimen of wild, rampant womanhood with a noble brown neck and nostrils that flared seductively every time she threw back her wonderful leonine head to laugh.

She wasn't ashamed of being a stripper, whilst I, to be honest, was absolutely thrilled about it. Nor was she too reticent when it came to supplying fine detail concerning her professional duties in the massage parlour.

'How would the man-in-the-street go about organising a massage from the likes of yourself?' I enquired.

'Private business, honey. Members only.' she drawled.

'Are you a trained masseuse?' I asked.

She narrowed her eyes and smiled wickedly. 'I get by.'

'Oh, I see.'

'I guess you do at that.'

'You have to . . . eh . . . do things?'

'You mean, over and above?'

'I suppose I do, if you don't mind me asking.'

'I don't mind.'

'Well?'

'Hand relief only, baby.'

'Of course. And what if the punters want to go . . . um . . . further?'

'Depends on if'n I like 'em or not.'

'What about, say, if someone like meself came in and . . . ah . . . wanted to go pretty far, so to speak?'

She laughed, and there went the nostrils again. 'You, honey! For you I'd go all the way . . . on the house!'

In my mind I could hear a distant hoot coming from the scum-coated waters of the Manchester Ship Canal.

It was the sound of my ship finally coming in.

I self-consciously crossed my legs and thanked God for what he had sent me.

Boyfriends of hand-relievers weren't permitted to enter the hallowed confines of the massage parlour section of the private club, but I was at liberty to roam the separate dingy striptease section, and habitually took my place at a small corner table amongst the baggy-eyed, grey-faced men who were seated at their own solitary small tables. Together we would silently watch the nubile Tina unveil her body three times a night to the strains of the tiredest band in the world.

Between sets she would join me for a convivial drink, and when she left to prepare for further disrobement, bedraggled strangers with bad breath would shuffle to my table, rustling money, and rasp furtive propositions into my ear.

They thought I was her pimp.

I waved them away, saying that we were engaged to be married.

If only the Christian Brothers could see me now.

They had prepared me well for this.

It couldn't last, of course.

Taking her home to meet my parents was not a realistic option. They may not have warmed to a prospective daughter-in-law who liked to meditate naked whilst hanging upside down from the trapeze bar that was a prominent fixture in her small flat. Nor might they have appreciated her habit of walking (yes, still naked) across the room on her hands, the white soles of her feet pointing gloriously heavenwards whilst she puffed at the Paki-Black joint clasped between her teeth. At times like this, one appreciated the glory that was gravity.

She was a one-off.

I stayed with her most nights for three or four exhausting weeks and, despite several invitations to move in permanently, I decided, though very tempted, not to accept. A still, small voice in my head warned of imminent disaster.

One late afternoon during breakfast, a very large black man walked in as if he owned the place.

He had used his own key.

She rushed to embrace him whilst I sat with a forkful of scrambled egg suspended halfway between plate and open mouth.

A guiltily rumpled bed stood in the corner.

I felt vulnerable.

At first, optimistically, I thought that he might have been a sibling, but quickly dismissed the notion when they practically devoured each other in a frantic, passionate, groping greeting.

They eventually disentangled.

'Well, hello, BABY!' she squealed.

He looked mean and shiny, swathed in black leather from head to toe . . . a dude.

'Who's he?' He jerked a bald head in my direction.

'Oh, just a guy.'

'You bangin' him?'

My heart stopped and cold sweat formed on my brow.

She threw back the great head that was so dear to me and laughed raucously.

'A girl's gotta do sumpin' to while away the time when you're not here!'

I was very afraid. This man would surely kill me. But he appeared not at all dismayed by the information he had just received.

I was very confused. On one level I was relieved to be in no immediate danger, but on another level, I was hurt that he seemed so unconcerned by what, by any civilised moral standards, was an unacceptable situation.

He clearly knew his way around the place and casually pulled open a cupboard door behind which both he and I knew lurked a bottle of beer.

He ripped the cap off with his teeth, took a manly slug, and grinned at Tina.

'Get him outta here,' he said. 'We gotta make up for lost TIME!' He rolled his tongue suggestively across his upper lip.

She smiled seductively, gave his buttocks a quick, vulgar squeeze and approached me in the matter-of-fact way that a dog-owner would busily approach her small, docile pet when it was time to go walkies.

'Time to go, honey. Party's over.'

I was ushered urgently towards the door, fork still in hand, capable only of making little whining sounds of timid protest. I complied more or less willingly though, thinking she was altruistically getting me out of there for my own protection, and to be truthful, I expected whispered assurances when we reached the door, and perhaps hurried arrangements made to meet later when she could explain this temporary blip and adopt a forward plan.

Came there none.

She left me outside the door like a dustbin.

I was still holding the fork.

That was it.

We never spoke to each other again.

Broken-hearted, I went back to the club once and watched her twice taking off her clothes, but she showed not a flicker of recognition and disappeared urgently when I tried to approach her.

I was just another punter.

I learnt then that there were alternatives to the White Man's Ways.

It was over for ever.

I slunk back to the hovel where myself and fellow band members were bivouacked and once again got used to eating baked beans served up on the filthy vinyl of old Frankie Vaughan long-playing records, and drinking beer downstairs with the landlady's husband who, after four pints, always insisted on showing us his war wound, which was an open, oozing, terrifyingly deep gash on the back of his lower right leg that for twenty years had refused to heal properly.

We tolerated this solely because the room was warm, and were forced to leave only when the old warrior reached the inevitable angry stage in his drinking where he would fulminate loudly against Rommel's arrogance in the desert, punctuating his complaints by smashing beer glasses on the tiled hearth.

Sighing, we would then trudge back upstairs to our unheated room, sometimes hearing on the landing above the nerve-jangling patter of fifty tiny feet on the thin linoleum – two of which were owned by the creepy landlady, the remaining forty-eight belonging to the twelve Scottish terriers that followed her in single file . . . a flea-ridden crocodile of the Devil's hair-balls.

We starved in Manchester for over a year until sinister forces scattered us to the four winds.

I think we first got scared when our trumpet player was asked to murder a local buildings inspector.

We were 'working' on the former site of a recently demolished factory. Our primary task was to clear the area to make way for a new building project, when we accidentally discovered an uncharted underground tunnel.

This news dismayed the site boss. He was bound by law to expend considerable time, energy and money ensuring that the vast tunnel was filled and sealed before he could sell the site on to the future builder.

Unfortunately the buildings inspector just happened to be there at the time and had gone down to have a look at this subterranean novelty.

Our trumpet player, dozing in a bulldozer, was approached by the site boss and asked to perform a certain manoeuvre just over the tunnel into which the buildings inspector had been lowered. The brick ceiling was in bad repair, and in danger of collapse. The trumpeter pointed this out. The site boss concurred and offered him £500 if he would nevertheless proceed with the operation and keep schtum afterwards.

Replying that he was a trumpeter and not an assassin, the offer was refused.

Things were never the same for us after that.

Accidents happened.

Our singer was hospitalised when an empty acetylene canister trundled out of nowhere and broke his leg.

Skinny but nimble musicians had to jump out of the trajectory of wrecking balls that swung too close for comfort.

Lorries inexplicably lurched in our direction.

Enough was enough. We decided to go our separate ways.

I sold my guitar to raise the fare home plus a little extra. Skipping my spartan lodgings via a moonlight flit, I caught the morning boat from Liverpool to Belfast. The others did the same, forgetting to say goodbye to our singer, still languishing penniless in hospital with his lower body in traction, comforted by the only friend he had in the whole of England, a Polish nurse who spoke little English. We knew he'd understand.

Two days later, back home in Stroke City where I'd started. Thinner but wiser.

Hello, Mum.

STAGE FOUR: *The Break for Glory*

This is a dangerous stage in the life of a musician. He is still a young man and has returned to the bosom of his family penniless after a considerable period of time spent largely in the company of drunks, crooks, hand relievers and potential or actual murderers.

He looks hard at his now-mature childhood friends and notes that most are happily married and making honest livings as carpenters, sparks and apprentice toolmakers.

To the man who is not serious about his music, this is a sign that he has taken the wrong path in life. He resolves to re-enter the mainstream of normal society by using his talents as a Routine Clerk to secure a clerical post in the Rates Office, Lane's Coal Office or any number of quill-wielding occupations that are open to him.

To a SERIOUS terminal musician, though, this is a time to merely regroup, refuel and otherwise get into good physical and mental shape, ready for a 'BREAK'.

Mine came in the form of a casual conversation with a musician friend who mentioned that a certain showband in Dublin was auditioning for a bass guitarist/vocalist.

The fact that I was neither of these in no way dampened my interest.

Dublin itself was the attraction. Once I got there I could become a bona fide guitar player again.

This would do in the mean time.

Anyway, I'd always had a sneaking regard for the bass guitar. What was it but the admittedly thicker bottom four strings of a conventional guitar? Just another form of plank-spanking. I could bluff that. Same principles.

As for singing? Anybody could sing. No special talent was required these days to croak out the nursery rhymes much loved by the paying punters.

And anyway, wasn't it a fact that most musicians regarded singers as having the brains of molluscs and treated them accordingly? How difficult could it be?

Singers usually reacted to this general disdain by developing uncontrollable piranha egos that demanded to be fed constantly.

I once played in a band that was fronted by a particularly nasty example of this flourishing species. He was partially deaf and wholly insane.

This is not a good combination.

Even normal, averagely sane singers like to hear themselves above the roar of the band, and this causes trouble enough, but congenital deafness exacerbates the problem.

It was my job to defend the volume control on the amplifier that powered the PA or Public Address System, as it was quaintly called in those days.

I was told to stand in front of it at all times, and if the singer made any attempt to interfere with the mechanism, I was empowered to use whatever force was deemed necessary to repel his advances.

Trouble came on the first night. He was singing Sam and Dave's 'Hold On, I'm Comin'', an intricate enough piece of vocal pyrotechnics involving, as it did, much simultaneously screaming brass and hooting saxophones.

I watched through hooded eyes as the veins in his neck bulged and his face turned crimson with effort.

I could hear his voice plainly enough above the racket, but it was obvious from the desperate glances he was shooting in my direction that he was not happy with the overall balance.

As the solo guitar weaved its dubious magic, he strode towards me with outstretched fingers probing for the volume control. I braced myself and defended the machine, feet planted firmly apart and guitar raised.

'Turn it up!' he cried. 'I can't hear myself!'

'That's cos you're deaf. It's fine, believe me,' I shouted.

'What was that?' he yelled back.

I gave up.

'Outta the way!' he screamed. 'Stand aside!'

'Hold fast,' I replied. 'I have my orders!'

'Turn the fucker up!' he demanded.

His hand flashed towards the volume knob. I had no choice. Arcing the neck of my stoutly constructed Fender guitar with some force, seasoned wood thwacked down upon flesh, bone and sinew.

He squealed with pain and fell over the drum-kit, clutching his throbbing wrist.

Wild-eyed with bloodlust, I wheeled on the spot, ready to dish out more of the same if he sprang back at me . . . I had become an animal.

Only then did I see the shocked expressions on the faces of two terrified girls who were standing in front of the stage holding on to each other for comfort, having witnessed this bestial act of aggression perpetrated in the name of showbusiness.

'What the fuck are YOU looking at?' I roared.

I had arrived.

I was now an all-round entertainer.

'St Louis down the Nat?'

This cryptic phrase came from the sly lips of a louche man who leaned from the driver's cab of the large streamlined coach that was illegally parked at the entrance to Amiens Street railway station in Dublin.

The vehicle belonged to the Chessmen Showband and the driver was observing the difficulty with which I was making my way down the station's stone steps, encumbered by a large, borrowed, wooden guitar case and other sundry unwieldy personal items.

At the bottom of the steps I had snagged my foot on the rim of a small pothole, and only the presence of a low wall prevented me from crashing to the ground.

I pulled myself together and approached the bandcoach that was there to meet me.

'St Louis down the Nat, huh?' the driver repeated, knowingly. 'Uh . . . Yes, I suppose so,' I answered, when what I really wanted to say was 'What the fuck are you talking about?'

He chuckled horribly and beckoned me aboard the otherwise empty vehicle.

I climbed up three steep steps, deposited my burden on what appeared to be seats commandeered from a commercial airliner, and marvelled at the symmetry and plushness of the vehicle's interior. Before I had time to settle, the engine roared into life and the craft lurched suddenly and recklessly into the teeth of a Dublin rush-hour traffic snarl. I held on grimly.

St Louis down the Nat, eh?

Only later did I discover that I had just heard my first example of 'Ben Lang', a peculiarly Dublin version of Cockney rhyming slang.

The driver had been alluding to my stumble in the street. 'St Louis' referred to my shoe, i.e., St Louis Blues = shoes (in this case singular); Nat = Nat King Cole = hole. *Ergo* St Louis down the Nat = shoe down the hole = possible unfortunate injury to fetlock.

Well, yes.

This was a new world peopled by musicians and ancillary personnel who spoke their own language.

Perched beside the driver, I stared in awe at the road ahead as he took tremendous driving risks whilst aiming a manic torrent of invective at other more hesitant drivers, only twenty per cent of which I could vaguely comprehend:

'Gerrup the yard (*translation: fuck off*), ya two ends of a nigger's jigger (*coloured man's sexual organ*)! Yer arse is parsley, ya bollix, ya (*mixed metaphor*)!

'Keep yer mincers (*eyes*) on the Lew Hoad (*road*), ya bum-bandit! SHIRT-LIFTER (*homosexual*)!!!

'Left hammer, left hammer (*specific driving manoeuvre*)!

Give 'er the holly, ya baaastard (*please accelerate*)!

'Wha! You wearing the beard (*form of oral sex*) or wha?

'Sweet Henry H. Christ (*mythical brother of Jesus*)!

'You'll have me in the bleedin' Dodder (*popular small local river flowing adjacent to the road*)!

'Dear fuckin' inconsolable sufferin' Mother a' Jaysus, will ya lookit that eejit (*self-explanatory*)!! Outta me way!!

'By the shirt of Matt Talbot (*local martyr*)! Shouldn't be on the bleedin' road at all! PIPE SMOKER (*yet another form of oral sex*)!!!

'Pox-doctor's clerk (*registrar of venereal diseases*)!!! Varney (*look at*) the jugs (*breasts*) on the charver (*patently loose woman*).

'Look at the thrupennies (*tits again, as in 'thrupenny bits'*) on dat!!!

'Check the gate (*female upper thighs exposed due to adoption of careless sitting position*)! Scotch Pegs (*legs*) up to her arse!

'Lookit! There's the jamjar (*car*) I've wanted since me hoop (*bodily orifice*) was the size of a shirt-button (*since early childhood*)! Look at the garden-hose (*nose*) on the aul wan (*elderly lady*)! Ya wouldn't want the change outta HER drawers (*underwear*)! Some Peggy Dell (*odour*) offa THEM!

'Wha! Look at the body on that Richard (*the Third = bird*)! I'd eat chips outta yer knickers! I'd use her shoite for tootpaste (*popular self-explanatory Dublin vulgarisms*)!'

Momentary silence.

'Jaysus, I'd love a jar (*alcoholic drink*)! I've a thirst I wouldn't swap for a fiver!

'Hey! Mind yourself! Watch that chiseller (*small child*), missus, or you'll be taking a mat (*flattened small child*) home! Are ya all right there, son?'

Pause.

'Are ya all right, I sez?' sez he, staring at me with wild eyes.

'Me? Oh . . . ahm . . . yes. I'm fine, thanks.'

Welcome to Dublin. Home to James Joyce, Yeats, O'Casey, Wilde and John Millington Synge; where language could still surprise. I knew that I was going to like this place.

And I did.

This was an important stage in my onward journey to wherever I would end up.

The Chessmen were, thankfully, a reluctant showband in that they did not, as some of the other poor bastards did, believe in what they were doing.

Originally what was described as a 'beat group', they were a five-piece outfit quite happily playing local sweaty blues clubs when, surprisingly, they were asked to make a record. The 'A' side was an instantly forgettable bowdlerisation of an obscure smutty Muddy Waters blues wail, and on the 'B' side, just for laughs, they had recorded a song called 'Michael Murphy's Boy', a satirical dig at the current popularity of ballads relating tearful tales of the Irish Diaspora a.k.a. the Scattering.

To their horror, the 'A' side was totally ignored and the 'B' side became a huge hit in the Irish charts.

Suddenly a hot property, they were advised to add brass and reed, go on the road as a showband and rake in large piles of money as rapidly as possible.

This they did, but their hearts weren't in it.

This suited me fine.

The band toured the country in some style, churning out populist crap but at the same time writing songs and experimenting with other musical forms which we would sometimes slip into our regular programme, to the general dismay of the blank-faced dancers, who (like their ballroom-dancing cousins) usually stopped automatically when they could no longer hear the Galway Wallop (the thudding snare-drum off-beat employed by country and western bands to ensure that the dancing tempo was embedded solidly in the confused heads of the twirling rustics). I was amongst cynics. That was where I was always happiest. I've found that earnestness and unquestioning enthusiasm make me depressed.

I got to know our roadie/driver well and we swapped cultural tales.

He told me about the man who lived next door to him who had to get rid of his ten-year-old Alsatian dog because, as I surely knew, Alsatians turn into wolves when they reach the age of eleven.

I told him about Stroke City and how I had once observed a banner, hoisted in a predominantly Catholic area during the Eucharistic Congress, which bore the legend: 'GOD BLESS OUR LORD'.

He didn't see anything unusual about that. He also told me about another man he knew who would spend the remainder of his days in a 'menatil institution' because he had waded in very cold water at Killiney Beach, just outside Dublin.

When I asked what permanent harm this could have caused, I was told that contact with the extremely cold water had caused the man's blood to rush straight to his head, rendering him permanently insane.

I, in turn, told him about the Stroke City youth who had been in court for kicking both an RUC man and his dog. The defendant was fined £150 for kicking the policeman and a further £200 for kicking the dog.

He didn't see anything unusual about that either.

Whilst travelling, I was his map-reader and road-sign-looker-out-for. He explained that he was too busy driving to be bothered with that sort of nonsense.

I soon discovered that I was assigned these duties solely because he was trying desperately to conceal the fact that he couldn't read.

It wasn't hard to spot. In restaurants he would study an often upside-down menu and, waiting until everyone else had ordered, would finally casually choose something he'd heard someone else mention. I admired his ingenuity. None of the other band members had twigged that he couldn't read. I didn't tell him I knew.

But his illiteracy sometimes caused problems.

'When are you going home next?' he once asked.

'Soon. Why?' I replied.

'Do you ever get Frenchies for the boys?' he whispered.

He was referring to the common-at-the-time practice of purchasing condoms in the north and flogging them surreptitiously to the prophylactically starved population of Catholic southern Ireland.

'Not as a rule. But I can get you some if you want,' I offered generously.

'Jazus, no!' he scoffed, glancing left and right.

He withdrew a crumpled piece of folded brown wrapping paper from his back pocket.

'I believe these are the boys for me! Get us a rake o' those.'

I was almost afraid to open the paper. When I did, I saw a single word scrawled in black marker pen. APHRODISIAC. Some smart bastard had written this down to wind him up.

'How much are they?' he asked, reaching his hand into his pocket.

'These might be hard to find. Not many chemists stock them. They're hot stuff. I'll have a go, though, and you can pay me when and if I get them.'

A less scrupulous person would have scraped the brand name from some Aspro tablets and sold them to him for a pound a pop.

I thought about doing so but hadn't the heart.

Probably would have perked up his sex life considerably, if indeed that was what he thought they were for. It was difficult to tell.

The band made records for which we had great hopes. One of the guys in the band had written a song called 'Billy Jones' about a boy who lived in a tree-house and urged young girls to visit him on a regular basis. I was called upon to sing this odd ditty and, on entering the recording studios to lay down the vocal, was stunned to find an entire symphony orchestra waiting to accompany me.

My first attempts at the song were distinctly tentative, tremulous and noticeably out of tune, causing members of the orchestra to emit small, embarrassed coughs.

The producer took charge of the situation and suggested that I relax more. To this end, he announced a short break and brought me next door to a pub, where I drank seven whiskeys in quick succession.

Returning flushed, I sang like a nightingale, and at the successful conclusion of the session was treated to a small smattering of applause from the distinguished members of the orchestra.

Such experience is invaluable.

A person learns the necessity of getting half-pissed before attempting anything important.

The record did not sell.

I enjoyed the next few years in Dublin, playing in a band that was popular in the cities but died in country areas. This was the natural order of things in a civilised world and I was having a good time, ensconced in a small, gloomy flat, eating too little, drinking too much and chasing a better class of woman.

The living was easy and I could afford to hop from one band to another, finally ending up with an outfit of a high musical standard, members of which spent considerable hours of rehearsal time mastering intricate five-part harmony vocals about which the dancers did not give a single fuck.

I regarded this as a sign of encouragement. I have always tried to live by the premise that any form of music disliked by the broad general public is intrinsically sound, meritorious and worth pursuing.

We were particularly excited about a pending tour of Canada and careful to stipulate that on no account would we play Irish clubs as a standard Irish touring band for Irish people.

We were assured that this would not be the case and that we would play regular club dates for ordinary Canadian folk . . . folk who would not break into floods of tears at the first strains of 'Danny Boy'.

Bolstered by these assurances, we set off excitedly and flew into Toronto, where we disembarked in high spirits after causing some consternation amongst other passengers by scattered bouts of over-boisterous behaviour occasioned by a surfeit of duty-free vodka.

Our first gig was at a club in Kingston, Ontario, where we were to perform for six nights. This was untold luxury for a band accustomed to bleary one-night stands and as we set up our equipment we already had our eyes peeled for the arrival of the incumbent waitresses. Pure animal instinct told us that those of us who snapped up the more attractive ones on the first night would, for the duration of the week, have first option on their carnal services if richer pickings were not to be found. A little basic insurance is always desirable.

We were relieved to discover that the manager of the club appeared not to be of Irish extraction by virtue of the fact that he completely ignored us, did not seem interested in which part of Ireland we were from, and had a normal-sized nose.

As the crowd filtered in, we kept a wary eye out for Irish expatriates. I had had previous experience of these in England but had been told that those in Canada and the USA were worse by far.

I had been told horror stories by other musicians who had toured northern America and been latched on to by lonely Irishmen who determinedly befriended them and insisted on getting the musicians out of bed at eight o'clock in the morning for tours of the immediate area, which usually included proud viewings of oil refineries, sewage plants, local irrigation schemes, tidal barriers, civic buildings, fish factories, canning plants and half-constructed highway flyovers.

I had been told of one case where a drummer appearing with a touring showband in Hamilton, Ontario, had been hounded cruelly by an Irish building worker from Cavan who insisted on teaching the musician how to mix cement the modern way.

After being pestered night and day by this uncomprehending pest, the desperate musician was forced to get rid of him by openly and lewdly propositioning the expatriate's extremely ugly Canadian girlfriend. It was the only way.

There seemed little chance of this in Kingston as we watched the punters filter into the club on our opening night. They appeared refreshingly half-human and many were smartly dressed in contemporary clothing.

We didn't mind being introduced as an Irish showband because, after all, I suppose that was what we were.

The deal was that we would play five half-hour sets, with half-hourly intervals in between, during the course of which we were told to 'work the room', i.e., table-hop, appear friendly, mingle seamlessly with the punters, thereby encouraging them to buy more drink.

Excitedly we trooped on-stage and played our first set. We had planned it carefully and included all the numbers on which we had worked so assiduously: a Beach Boys song with intricate five-part vocal harmony, a little modern jazz, a Mose Allison blues, an a cappella version of 'Smoke Gets in Your Eyes', an accomplished version of a Swingle Singers' track from the album *Jazz Sebastian Bach*. We were cookin'.

Ah! Wasn't it great to play civilised music in a civilised country and not have to worry about the limited sensibilities of rough, stubbly bastards wearing blue suits with brown shoes who demanded nothing more than a primitive rhythmic thump to facilitate noisy buck-lepping about on a paraffin-oil-soaked floor, grimly clutching the muscular bodies of beehived, dropped-arsed dragons whose upper thighs seemed permanently situated below their mottled knees.

The Canadian audience listened politely.

At the end of our set, we filed off to a strange silence and, never for a moment interpreting this lack of appreciative applause as anything other than natural reticence, trooped into the band room to towel down in preparation for our first 'working of the room'.

Our manager was already there, lazily reading the *Toronto Star*.

'How did it go?' he enquired uninterestedly.

'Great!' someone said. 'I think we surprised them. A bit quiet, though, I thought they were. The crowd, y'know?'

We heard an urgent knock on the dressing-room door.

The manager of the club bustled in. 'What the fuck are you guys playing at?' he demanded, sucking forcefully on a small cigar.

'Something wrong?' our manager ventured.

'Are you trying to empty my club? This is a pub, for fuck's sake. What kinda shit is that you're playing out there? This isn't the fuckin' Albert Hall, London, England! Where's the Irish music? Liven the fucker up! People want to be goddamn entertained! They're falling asleep out there! Half the room isn't even drinking.'

A cardinal sin. Nothing worse than a teetotal room.

'Maybe they're just enjoying the music?' suggested a brave soul amongst us.

'So how come some of them are leaving? Play your Irish stuff! That's what they came to hear.'

'We don't do any,' I chirped.

He glared at me over the glowing tip of his evil-smelling cigar.

'Ya don't do any what?'

'We don't do Irish music.'

'You will if you wanna get paid,' was his significant reply.

At this, our manager immediately sprang to life and managed to calm down the angry Canadian impresario by explaining that there had indeed been a misunderstanding; that, regrettably, we did not at present include an Irish element in our programme; that we would play a programme consisting entirely of Irish music from tomorrow night on; that we would apologise to the present audience tonight and ask them to bear with us for the inconvenience we had caused them; that we would rehearse all day tomorrow and all the days after that; and do you think that would be acceptable, sir, and will you still pay us after we do all that and three bags full, sir?

Fuck me, I thought. It's the same all over the world.

Is there no escape?

The night passed uneasily and we awoke depressed and

early the next morning to spend the entire day gloomily rehearsing old leprechaun chestnuts: 'The Bold O'Donahue', 'Danny Boy', 'Boolavogue', 'The March Hare', 'The Siege of Ennis', 'Does Your Mother Come from Ireland', 'Galway Bay' and, sadly, 'The Hokey-Cokey'.

C'est la guerre.

But there was light at the end of the tunnel.

After four weeks of this torture in various Canadian towns, our faithful manager absconded suddenly with the bulk of our money, leaving the door of his motel room swinging gently in the wind.

We were marooned and penniless, with no prospects.

Having little or no choice and tiny open mouths to feed, the three married members of the band fled home to face their familial responsibilities, leaving the four single lads (including me) who had nothing of any substance to go back to.

We decided to brazen it out as a small group and rapidly procured a dodgy agent, who immediately fixed us up with a series of gigs in less than salubrious pubs and clubs located in undesirable urban areas and remote mining towns where men were men and we weren't.

Some of them were interesting enough, though. We once played a small, sparsely populated town near the American–Canadian border. One afternoon, having a little time to kill, I took a brisk walk and ended up having a beer in a bar on the outskirts of town. The bartender wanted to know where I was from.

'I'm Irish.'

'Don't get many Irish around here. Plenty Indians though.'

My ears pricked up.

'Indians?'

'Yeah, from the reservation.'

'I've never met a real Indian,' I confided.

'Count yourself lucky,' he snorted. 'They're ornery.'

I would be ornery too if I was cooped up in a reservation by the White Eyes. Northern Ireland was difficult enough to endure.

'What do you mean, ornery?' I asked.

'They get mean when they drink.'

'Doesn't everybody?'

'Not after two glasses of beer they don't. An Indian's digestive system can't process alcohol. Something to do with his stomach juices. Alcohol goes straight to his brain. Give 'em a pint of beer and watch out!'

'I can't believe that,' I said.

'OK. Come here Thursday afternoon and find out.'

'Why Thursday?'

'That's when they get their welfare cheques. They always come in here to cash 'em.'

What a load of superior bollocks, I thought. No wonder the Indians hated us. That was what was wrong with this world. Too much stereotyping and misinformation. I got enough of that at home.

Thursday afternoon came. I was there at 2 p.m.

'What time do they come in?' I asked.

'Set your seat-belt for three thirty,' said the bartender.

In they filed at the appointed time. They were a sullen bunch and I was disappointed to find that they were dressed in regular clothes, although some wore hats adorned with the occasional feather. Token feather, I thought sadly.

But there was no mistaking their sallow skin and noble profiles. These were Indians, all right.

Cheques were cashed and pitchers of beer produced. The Indians sat around tables in groups of six or seven, quietly sipping from half-pint glasses.

The bartender winked at me and tapped his nose with his index finger.

I didn't like him very much and felt I shouldn't have been there. After about ten minutes I noticed the noise level in the room rise considerably.

The Indians had suddenly become very animated, and one or two were on their feet, shouting angrily.

Another Indian walked towards the bar, stumbled and began laughing very loudly.

Fuck me, I thought. That Indian's pissed. He's only been here ten minutes.

Soon they were all drunk, singing weird songs and falling about the place. I was amazed.

I turned round to talk to the bartender and noticed that an older Indian had taken a chair next to mine. He appeared sober but did not look at me. He had a great hooked nose, a full head of long white hair tied in a ponytail, and a sorrowful expression. He was nursing a rye whiskey. I began to get nervous. If two glasses of beer made the young bucks crazy, what would whiskey do to an older brave?

He seemed in control, though, so I decided to attempt some form of communication. I leaned over and offered him a cigarette.

He ignored me completely, fished out his own cigarettes and lit one.

Well, that's a snub. I gave up.

At this point the bartender came over and I ordered another drink.

I felt a tap on my shoulder. It was the old Indian.

'Where you from?' he asked haltingly.

I was surprised.

'Ireland,' I answered.

'Ahhhhh,' he said. His voice trailed away.

'What tribe are you?' I asked.

'Never mind. We're the same.'

'Who is? Who's the same?'

'You and I,' he said.

'Are we?'

'We both suffer indignity under white man.'

'But I thought I was white.'

'No, you're Irish. I know a song,' he said. 'You know it too.'

He stood up unsteadily and I realised that he was pissed, too.

I stood up.

Who knows what a stranger would have thought had he

entered this bar and witnessed the spectacle of an Irishman and a Chippewa elder, arms wrapped around each other's shoulders, lustily bawling the anthem known to the world's oppressed:

'WE SHALL OVERCOME, WE SHALL OVERCOME, WE SHALL OVERCOME, SOME DAY-Y-Y-Y-Y!'

But I digress.

Our new agent had flown the coop.

Fate then intervened.

During a week's engagement at a scabrous pub in a town with bad air called Peterborough, I noticed, standing at the bar, a man who didn't look as if he should be there at all.

He was tall, slim, with a mane of blond hair, and he wore a trendy full-length, snugly fitting, expensive leather greatcoat and hand-crafted cowboy boots that poked out from a tasty pair of skin-tight, stone-washed Levi jeans.

He stood out from the regular gruff patrons who were mostly check-shirted, baggy-arsed, squat, beer-guzzling, white-trash thugs from the local granite quarry.

He looked somehow vaguely familiar.

He was there again the following night and I was further intrigued by the fact that he didn't drink or speak to anybody and appeared to concentrate very heavily on the band.

He was listening to us.

I didn't know why.

We were just getting used to being completely ignored.

He was there again on our final night (Saturday) and, as I was routinely ordering an anaesthetising double rye whiskey at the bar, he approached in a mannerly fashion.

'Hi! My name is Dwayne English,' he announced in a rolling Texan drawl. To my surprise and amazement, it transpired that he was a fairly famous rock drummer whom I had recently seen in a notoriously chaotic film called *Mad Dogs and Englishmen*. This film was the stuff of legend, a celluloid record of drug abuse and wild times during an American tour undertaken by a groggy Joe Cocker, a crazed

Leon Russell, a demure yet stunned Rita Coolidge and a variety of musicians in various stages of moral and physical disintegration.

I admired the film greatly and immediately warmed to Mr English, who seemed a reformed, reasonable and civilised soul.

I was amazed to see him. What was he doing in this sink-hole?

He told me that he had recently joined a reincarnation of a rock 'n' roll outfit called Ronnie Hawkins and the Hawks. The band was living and rehearsing at Hawkins' large ranch, which was just a few miles outside of town.

When I asked him who Hawkins was, he told me that he was a singer from Arkansas whose previous band of Hawks had been purloined by Bob Dylan some time ago and were now called The Band.

Big stuff, thought I, increasingly interested.

My eyes popped as he continued.

He said that the new Hawks didn't have a bass guitarist yet, and although some people from New York were due to fly in for a try-out, he thought I'd have as good a chance as any of them, and would I care to audition for the band?

Of all the ginjoints in all the world.

Would I care to audition for the band?

Would a chimp chomp on a banana?

Would a squirrel eat nuts?

Fuckin' right, I would.

I'd been waiting long years for this break.

When I pushed him for more detail, he revealed that the band was shaping up well but resting at the moment until the line-up was finalised, adding that the past week had been a bit of a party week, with a few guests dropping by.

When pushed further, he intimated that John Lennon and Yoko Ono had stayed at the ranch recently, and that Kris Kristofferson was still there, drinking for America.

I couldn't believe what I was hearing and would have doubted this man's credentials had I not recognised him from the film. He was kosher.

These men obviously moved in rarefied circles.

John Lennon and Yoko fuckin' Ono!!

Mr English told me that Mr Hawkins had approved the idea of the proposed audition and there was no need to bring any equipment because everything I needed would be there, and would I find it convenient to be picked up in front of this pub tomorrow morning (Sunday) at 10 a.m.?

I certainly would.

Bidding him adieu, I was faced with the task of concealing my excitement from members of my own band.

I couldn't tell them about this! They would spontaneously combust due to jealousy, begrudgery and spleen-bile. Furthermore, marvellous career opportunity or not, I would still be vilified roundly for being the first rat to scuttle down the hawser.

We were due to move camp next day anyway, so it was relatively easy for me to invent a reason to be discovered in an unaccustomed perpendicular state at the hellish hour of nine o'clock on a Sunday morning. Having spun the yarn that I had some concubine or other to see and would team up with them again on Monday, there was little chance of being observed as I stood outside the prearranged rendezvous point.

It was early October, and the harsh Canadian winter wind had little difficulty penetrating the folds of my cheap Marks & Spencer gaberdine coat. My teeth chattered as the unfamiliar, crisp, fresh morning air conspired to surround me.

It was raining steadily and my shoes leaked.

What if I failed the audition?

Why wasn't I nervous?

Was it always this cold outside motel rooms?

As I sought answers to these questions, a large, sleek Rolls Royce slithered to a halt, the driver's window purred elegantly down and a scruffy, bearded man wearing a faded denim shirt shouted something in my direction.

Something was wrong. This man had a look of madness in his eye that did not sit easily with the stewardship of such a magnificent machine. He had probably stolen it.

He shouted again.

'Are you the man?' he screamed heartily.

'I don't know,' I replied, edging away. A fellow had to be careful in a foreign country.

'Are you Dwayne's man?' he enquired, more contained.

I noticed he had that peculiar flat Canadian accent that always reminded me of urban Ulster tones. Not for nothing was Toronto often referred to as West Belfast.

Fuck! I thought. This car's for me!

'Yes, I think I am,' I replied hesitantly, only then noticing the 'hawk in flight' motif that adorned the side of the car. Nice touch.

'I'm Rick,' he said. 'Jump in.'

Rather embarrassed, I walked over to the front passenger door and placed my hand on the finely turned handle.

'No, no!' he cried. ' Ride in back. Live a little.'

I did as I was bid.

I had never been chauffeured in a Rolls Royce before.

It felt good.

'We're going to Toronto!' Rick shouted over his shoulder, as the great craft pulled out from the kerb.

I was confused. Toronto was at least 150 miles away.

'Aren't we going to some kind of farm or ranch?' I enquired.

'Change of plan. Big party in TO tonight. OK?'

TO was OK with me. I never had been a party-pooper and didn't intend to start now.

We sailed along in silence and, such was the luxurious nature of the Roller's interior, I soon fell asleep. I hadn't been up this early in years.

Consciousness returned as the Rolls lurched to a halt at the end of a long driveway in front of a large, well-appointed mansion.

Rick leaped out and opened my door.

'Chocks away, matey!' he laughed. 'Is that English enough for you to feel at home?'

'You can be as English as you want to be. I'm Irish.'

A surly enough comment, but it appeared important at the time. Got things straight from the off.

We entered a great empty hallway and I followed Rick towards a large, pillared doorway from beyond which could be heard the buzz of excited conversation.

We found ourselves in an opulent room with elaborate wallpaper and ceiling frescos depicting naked cherubs. In the centre of the highly polished wooden floor was a white grand piano, and encircling it, lounging on vast, comfortable and expensive cushion-strewn sofas, was an eclectic mix of people.

There were conventional hippies, sober-suited bank-manager types, nymphettes, stern-costumed, flint-eyed women, dandys, fops, artistic, Byronesque, worried-looking young men, washed-out women who probably wrote poetry too, a man of the cloth, pale musicians, a number of free-range children and two scampering, panting dogs.

I had never seen a gathering quite like this before.

I noticed the tall figure of Dwayne English bearing down on me and I welcomed the sight of a familiar face.

'Made it, boy!' he beamed. 'Come and meet the Hawk.'

He led me across the room towards a large, avuncular man wearing a white stetson who was holding court amid a ruck of giggling women of varying shapes and sizes. He was gesticulating furiously as he related some tale or other. We hovered on the fringe of the company, waiting for an opportune moment to present ourselves.

The Hawk was in full flight. 'They told me they were on what they called a ma-cro-bi-ot-ic diet, eatin' only nuts and grains and stuff, and talked about Yin and Yang and horseshit like that. I said, "Fine, each to his own. It ain't my way but good luck to ya." Anyways, later on that night, 'bout four o'clock in the mornin', I couldn't sleep and took myself off for a short walk thinkin' everybody had turned in for the night. I saw a light on in the kitchen and thought, 'Sheeet, don't nobody turn off lights at night no mo?' I went inside and heard voices. I crept up to the kitchen door and guess what I saw? Only John and

Yoko standing by the open ice-box eating chicken, roast beef and anything else they could lay their hands on . . . ravenous, they were, like wild dogs! They were surprised to see me. What could I do! 'John,' I said. 'I've been on that ma-cro-bi-ot-ic diet all my life and didn't fuckin' know it!'

He beamed broadly, and the company tittered.

'Whatcha got there, Dwayne?'

'It's the Irish kid, Ronnie.'

'What's yo' name, boy?'

I told him.

'I'll just call you "Irish", OK?'

Well, it wasn't really OK, but now was not the time to make a stand.

'Make yourself at home, Irish. Have a drink!'

He turned away and resumed his role as raconteur.

Dwayne steered me towards the bar and introduced me to a very attractive lady from Nashville who was married to a man prominent in the music business. She shook my hand and held on to it long enough for me to know that it was going to be downhill from there on.

Day turned into night, and I mixed freely, drank heavily and thoroughly enjoyed myself.

As the night wore on, the crowd thinned, leaving just a dozen or so diehards shooting the breeze. I was very drunk and remember little, other than the telling of preposterous tales about Ireland to a seemingly interested but admittedly captive audience.

I woke up next morning with a pounding head to discover that I was not alone. Beside me lay a very attractive lady from Nashville who was married to a man prominent in the music business.

There was a gentle rap on the door and a cheery female voice piped, 'Last call for breakfast, hear? Chow-time!'

It was eleven o'clock in the morning. I had to be out of there by at least early afternoon to link up with the lads. Jesus! I was supposed to be playing that night at a new gig 300 miles from here! And I still had an audition to do!

I crept out while my new companion lay supine, and wandered sheepishly downstairs to a surprisingly normal breakfast scene in the large farmhouse kitchen.

Around the table sat a cheerful Hawk, his pretty wife and a number of small children. I felt awful.

'Sleep good, Irish?' said the Hawk.

'Yes, pretty good,' I replied.

'I'm not surprised. You drank all ma whiskey!'

'Sorry about that.'

My stomach heaved at the sight of a plate of English muffins that the Hawk's wife now placed before me.

Everybody ate in a comfortable silence.

I thought of the lady lying upstairs in bed and felt thoroughly ashamed that I had let myself down.

Time to speak. 'I must apologise for getting a bit tiddly last night. It's not like me.'

'Sure it is,' said the Hawk. 'No need to apologise.'

'Er...I think I may be a little behind schedule. I'm supposed to be in Northern Ontario this afternoon. When would you like me to ... ah ... do the audition?'

The Hawk gave a great snort.

'You did that last night, Irish.'

I must've been drunker than I thought.

'I don't seem to recall doing an audition,' I stuttered.

'You don't understand, Irish. I leave it up to Dwayne to judge whether or not your chops are up to playing with the band. He says they are, so I believe him. I'm only interested in finding out what kinda guy you are. Quickest way I know how to find out what a guy's like is to fill him up with whiskey and see how he jumps. Saves time. Why give a guy a job only to find out three weeks later that we can't get along? Get 'im drunk, I say. You see the real guy straight away. You're no saint, but then again, I ain't lookin' for no saint. You'll do.'

I'll do?

'Does that mean that you want me in the band?'

'It's up to you. I know you already got commitments. You're in if you want. Sort out your affairs and come back to me with an answer. But don't take too long. I gotta know within two weeks. I'll be at the Nickelodeon in Toronto. Rick'll take you wherever you want to go.'

Take me due north, Rick! And don't spare the lash!

After a long, ecstatic journey in the back of the Hawkmobile, I arrived at the sulphur-mining town of Sudbury. The foul air bit into my lungs as I descended from the Rolls Royce to greet my grey-faced fellow Gaels, who were wearily unloading our equipment from an ice-encrusted van into another faded pub.

To a man they stared in wonder at the magnificent machine, blanching at the apparition of my regal emergence from its stylish innards.

'Well, it's like this, lads . . .

STAGE FIVE: What Went Wrong?

I first realised that something was wrong when I began to look forward to seeing people I didn't know who played in other touring Irish showbands.

As a member of the legendary Hawks, one of the finest rock 'n' roll bands in the country, I had become a role model for my fellow Irish musicians, living proof that there was a God after all. One of their own who had come good.

During our periodic stints at the Nickelodeon, showband musicians would arrange to come to the gig on a night off. The 'Hawks' were a flamboyant outfit. My friends would marvel at the top-hatted and bearded Doctor Fingers on virtuoso rock 'n' roll piano. Jaws would drop at the pyrotechnics of guitar wunderkind Dave Van Deusen. Celtic feet would tap to the intricate but earthy beat of heart-throb drummer Dwayne. Note would be taken of Ronnie Hawkins' almost superhuman stage presence and showmanship. Ears would pin back at the primeval roar of a band rehearsed to within an inch of its life, gloriously firing on all cylinders, and there, in the middle of it all . . . was me. A dog's-arse like themselves.

It gave them hope.

Like as not, famous faces would be seen amongst the audience. Such was Ronnie's legendary reputation that it was not unusual to see a table cleared and made ready for the expected Clint Eastwood or Bob Dylan party.

Kris Kristofferson, then just about the biggest name in the business, was a regular when in town. He drank Bushmills whiskey like a man trying to enter the *Guinness Book of Records.*

It wasn't unusual to find oneself having a beer and man-to-man chats with the likes of Frank Zappa, Gordon Lightfoot or members of current global hit band Blood, Sweat and Tears.

And, oh look, there's George Peppard!

Rock 'n' roll tinged with a little Hollywood fairy-dust attracts a fairly impressive retinue of hangers-on, and in this case there certainly was a surfeit of glamorous high- and low-life.

Drugs were not uncommon. Beautiful, immoral women were not just ten a penny, but absolutely free of charge.

This was a happening place. My showband friends naturally didn't feel part of it and normally just observed the proceedings huddled self-consciously around a faraway table. Way out of their depth.

Trouble was, I discovered that I was happiest sitting with them, soon realising that they were usually by far the most natural, normal and well-adjusted people in the room.

Something was wrong.

Gradually I also came to the conclusion that perhaps there was more to life than a schnozzleful of cocaine and the company of vacuous friends who would confess to me their darkest and most private secrets one day, and fail to recognise me twenty-four hours later.

Nor was I much encouraged by getting to know so-called big names in the music business, a surprisingly large majority of whom were Walking Wounded.

Most were desiccated by alcohol, drugs or a combination of both, and some had weaknesses bordering on the psychopathic.

I found out that a person can get away with almost anything if rich and famous enough. This, of course, is nothing new, but it's a different matter when one sees, as I once did, an eighteen-year-old girl crying alone at a party after being raped and beaten by a 'household name' who was sublimely untroubled by the fact that what he had just done would have meant a fifteen-year jail sentence for an ordinary mortal.

It gets personal for me when others seem unconcerned.

Hey, it's a party! Didn't she know the score?

I craved the company of ordinary people.

Maybe I just wasn't cut out for this sort of thing after all. Of course there was more to life than this. But what?

I could do something else, couldn't I?

I was still a relatively young man, in non-rock 'n' roll terms. Hadn't I recently developed an interest in playing classical guitar, and hadn't I always been fascinated by archaeology? Maybe I could split the difference and become a Classical Archaeologist? Anything was possible. Not too late to start again?

After a year, I decided I didn't want to be a professional rock musician any more.

I realised that it *was* too late for me.

Life would be too short.

I'd had enough. Time to return to Stroke City before the terminal Stage Six kicked in.

Oh, and . . .

STAGE SIX: What the Fuck Are Those Young Guys Playing? Jesus! That's Not Music! It's Just NOISE!!!!

No thanks.

DUBLIN DAYS:
A POSTSCRIPT

'I'M NOT AN entertainer! I'm an ACTOR!!!'

The stentorian voice seemed to flutter the flock wallpaper that clung tenuously to the crumbling walls of the hotel lounge, startling a number of the inmates. But to regulars it signalled business as usual.

The owner of the booming voice was on his feet glaring fiercely at a frightened American tourist with whom, until this moment, he had been having what appeared to be a pleasant and civilised conversation.

The thespian was a small, tubby, dapper, elderly man with a powdered face and a shiny, blue-black wig, the extremity of which stuck out jaggedly where the fat neck emerged from his shirt collar, a wig that seemed to change colour alarmingly at any sudden movement of his head.

It was whispered locally that underneath the disastrous hairpiece grew a perfectly normal, full head of hair but nobody could prove it other than by wrenching the covering from his skull.

His face burned red with anger, a condition that did not noticeably improve as he rapidly downed a final, medicinal large whiskey in one noisy gulp. He turned from the flustered American and fixed an angry eye on the wispy-haired, elephantine man alongside him who had the imperial nose of a Roman senator and the body of Charles Laughton.

'Come! Hilton!!' he roared and flounced towards the exit,

his extraordinary head held remarkably high, given his distinct lack of stature.

The elephant man sighed wearily, brushed the cigarette ash from his cavalry twill trousers and followed stiffly in the wake of the angered party.

I sighed with pleasure as I watched Michael MacLiammoir and Hilton Edwards disappear into the night, bitching and squabbling as they minced towards O'Connell Street.

Michael MacLiammoir, the last of the great actor-managers, legendary co-founder (with Hilton) of the Gate Theatre Company in Dublin. Playwright, painter, author, discoverer of Orson Welles, one of the few Englishmen who spoke fluent Irish, the finest actor of his generation, the definitive Iago to Welles's stunning celluloid Othello. He was Oscar Wilde incarnate. A man given to extremes of behaviour, more than capable of causing a public scene when friendly Americans asked how long he had been in the entertainment business.

He was an ACTOR . . . There was a difference.

And then there was Hilton (also English). A gifted actor and producer, he was Michael's long-suffering companion and lover; the voice of reason that kept MacLiammoir's tempestuous genius on an even keel.

Two Englishmen who had become more Irish than the Irish themselves. Refugees from the 'mainland' and standard-bearers of a culture that wasn't theirs.

I treasured the moment and knew that I would never see men like these again.

They were wonderful; and Dublin was a wonderful city.

The time was the late sixties and I was in Groome's Hotel doing what I did best . . . watching the actors.

It was a small establishment situated on Cavendish Row directly opposite the hallowed Gate Theatre itself, not too far from the rival Abbey Theatre, which was known for staging predominantly pigs-in-the-kitchen 'Oirish' plays as opposed to the former's more progressive approach.

Not for nothing were the Gate and Abbey theatres referred

to as, respectively, Sodom and Begorrah.

Groome's Hotel is gone now. Until recently the site was occupied by the Kentucky Fried Chicken people, but in those pre-fast-poultry days it was a school of excellence for actors, agents, hellraisers, racing types, tellers of tall tales, flimflam men and terminal drinkers.

I was sitting with our trombonist who was afraid to drink because when he did he couldn't stop, and when he couldn't stop he got very drunk and when he got drunk he was in the habit of lurching into the street determined to hitch-hike home. Not to his home here in Dublin, which was a small, untidy flat that we both shared, but home to Belfast – his yearned-for point of geographical and spiritual origin.

And, if allowed to proceed, he sometimes made it across the heavily fortified border, only to return repentant the next day, muttering words to the effect that he didn't know what had come over him.

I had long since given up trying to understand why alcohol regularly set him off on this lemming-like trek and put it down to some preternatural character flaw over which he had little control.

I had no such urges.

I was happy here. Looking at the actors.

I had an arrangement with the night porter, a small, shabby, beaten man who had seen too much . . . a man who had touched his forelock in deference so often that his right hand seemed permanently glued to his forehead.

He was the man who had to contend with the likes of Peter O'Toole and Richard Harris roaring in from the street, trailed by a retinue of scarlet women and philistine men who would settle in the lounge and demand vast amounts of drink to be ferried in from stage right.

He was the man who whistled tunelessly as the lounge furniture was eventually hurled about the room to loud cackling and menacing whoops. His mission was not to put a stop to this destruction, but quietly to assess the damage, an estimate of which he carefully entered into a little book that dangled from his dark-blue apron.

Subsequently a bill would be presented which, I am led to believe, would be settled without rancour in the harsh light of day.

Other equally bright or lesser representatives of the acting profession, would turn up as the night progressed, transforming this quiet central hotel into a nightmare Rabelaisian parade of mature men engaged in a fruitless search for their personalities.

Maybe that's why they were actors.

During occasional turgid conversations with the night porter, I would sometimes ask what he thought of these rampant males who abused the premises in his care without thought or apology.

With a shrug of his shoulders he would reply: 'Well, they're not like ordinary people, are they? They're more sensitive than you or I. And you have to think of the tremendous pressure they have to endure in the public eye.'

In my bollocks.

I could do with a little of that pressure, I thought, eyeing the gorgeous women who were hanging on to every slurred word emanating from the crumpled form of a well-known film actor who had vomit on his shoes.

I was under pressure too.

Under pressure five nights a week, travelling long distances over neglected Irish roads, fellow band members huddled together for warmth, entombed in small, dangerously overloaded Ford Transit vans, comforted only by bottles of Jack Daniels lifted from a crate which, unlike any of the human occupants, regally occupied a single seat of its own.

Arriving at the usual squat, brick dance-hall, the band would tumble out of the van and groggily set up the stage equipment, usually under the unforgiving and penetrating gaze of the rat-faced proprietor, prior to being summoned to consume the mandatory bad meal, usually served up by a sniffy woman of a certain age with a serious physical deformity. Salads were popular (why waste heat cooking for these ungrateful bastards?), consisting of a wisp of lettuce and a slice of Gulag Archipelago Ham so thin that it resembled the negative print of a high-altitude photograph of some large Eastern Bloc city.

Sometimes, however, we stumbled upon riches in unlikely quarters.

Once, finding ourselves in the wilds of Connaught and suitably refreshed after a meal similar to the above, we, as a body, decided to take a little collective air and, having some time to kill, visit a local hostelry.

A passing cyclist braving the stiff wind was asked to point us in the direction of the nearest pub.

'There's no pub around here,' he shouted over his shoulder. Then added cryptically: 'But you'll get a drink in Farrelly's, two miles down in that direction.'

A wavering hand pointed due south.

There were a number of puzzling elements contained in these apparently conflicting pieces of information, but I didn't worry too much. I was used to hearing things that I didn't fully understand and could perhaps be considered past caring about almost anything.

Maybe I'd been on the road too long.

Proceeding bumpily in the direction indicated, we did indeed come across a clutch of buildings, one of which had a sign without, bearing the Farrelly legend.

The building appeared derelict: wide doors clenched shut, no visible lights from within, and a wooden window shutter flapping noisily in the wind. We half-expected to meet a tumbleweed careering down the middle of the road but were heartened by the sight of a scrawny, moth-eaten hound lying on its side at Farrelly's gable wall, the gale mercilessly whipping its exposed undercarriage.

The presence of the cur was a good omen, indicating that the dog's master could be within the confines of the building, drinking whiskey.

Explorers bravely bent against the raging storm, we approached the front door with some curiosity and were mildly surprised to find a small, neat, handwritten note tacked to its surface, beside a large protruding key.

The note read thus:

THIS IS NOT A PUBLIC HOUSE. HOWEVER, IF YOU WISH TO VISIT, PLEASE TURN KEY AND ENTER.

Having little choice but to follow these terse instructions, I turned the key and entered a gloomy hallway that led to a door on the left from behind which came the sound of muffled talk.

I peeped round the inner door to find, under a dangerously low ceiling, a small room crammed with dowdy men. Conversation ceased and scores of rheumy eyes stared at me.

I uttered a tentative 'Hello' and to a man they turned away, resuming their various mumbled conversations. An attractive girl made her way across the dirt floor, head stooped to avoid the low wooden roof beams. She had dark, wild hair and the unblemished alabaster skin of the innocent.

'Come in, then,' she snapped, and moved away to speak gently to a wizened man who sat on the edge of a wooden bench clutching a pint glass of Guinness. She removed a pipe from his pocket. As she did so, his mouth automatically gaped open, revealing blackened stumps of teeth that reminded me of a burnt-out forest. She placed the pipe firmly in his open maw and lit it with a long match.

He gave the pipe a few Popeye puffs and it functioned to his evident satisfaction.

We edged our way forward and stood in the centre of the floor. Contrary to the information we had gleaned from the note on the door, this seemed very much like a public house to me. The bar-top was the usual grocer's counter and optics could be observed supporting upside-down bottles of regular spirits. There were also hand-pumps for the dispensation of stout and sundry bottles of beer stood to attention on the shelves. All seemed shipshape, albeit a tad worn and mildewed.

I gently pushed my way through to the bar counter.

There was, of course, no one behind it.

I stood patiently for a while, drumming my fingers on the bar-top, whilst the old man who had just had his pipe lit moved slowly around the corner of the bar until he was behind the counter seemingly adopting a serving stance. 'Right!' I shouted. 'Could I have five pints of stout, a large Bush and a Monk by the neck?'

The old man stared at me blankly and slowly turned away. The girl was instantly by my side.

'What do you think you're doing?' she hissed sharply.

'I was . . . ah . . . ordering a drink,' I replied.

She pointed towards the street. 'Didn't you read the note on the door? This is no pub!' She tossed her head on the word 'pub', causing me to suddenly fancy her a great deal.

'Well,' I said. 'Excuse me for being so forward, but it certainly looks like a pub, feels like a pub, smells like a pub, and, forgive me, but aren't those men standing about drinking alcohol, drinking alcohol? There's drink on all the shelves, whiskey in the jars, vodka and gin in the bottles, hand-pumps on the bar, glasses on the counter. Call me presumptuous, but that's a pub where I come from!'

'It is not!' she stated emphatically. 'Who are ye people anyway?'

'We're musicians. We're appearing tonight in Whatyoumaycallit up the road.'

'Are ye sure?' she enquired suspiciously.

I turned to my trusty trombonist. 'Jimmy. Show her your credentials.'

Jimmy immediately produced his trombone mouthpiece from a trouser pocket, a weighty metallic article that he kept handy on his person at all times for the purpose of adding authority to his fist in case he was forced to punch somebody.

'Right,' she said. 'I believe yese.'

'It's OK,' I said. 'What's going on here?'

'It's me father's pension,' she whispered. 'He thought he wouldn't be granted his pension if he still had the pub when he reached the age of entitlement, so he closed it down and gave up the licence, but he wanted to carry on business as usual 'cos he missed it and wanted to put one over on the Government 'cos he worked hard all his life and why shouldn't he get a pension 'cos it's no skin off their noses and didn't he deserve it 'cos even those who haven't a shoe on their foot and never did a tap of work in their lives are getting the pension and why shouldn't he benefit like the rest of them, so he kept this place going in his own way but it's not the same 'cos we're not a pub but it's as near to a pub as a pub can get without actually bein' a pub at all, so officially we're not a pub at all so we're not. We're just not!'

She stood breathless and her chest heaved.

I was falling in love, but now was not the time to tell her.

'So, we can't order a drink then?' I said.

'No, you can't. But I can ask you if you'd like something to refresh you.'

'And if you ask me that, what happens if I reply that I would be very refreshed if you brought me five pints of stout, a large Bush and a Monk by the neck?'

'Well, in that case, I'll enter the private parlour behind the bar. I will then eventually make my way to an optic from which I will extract a large Bush. As time progresses I will then gather about me person five pints of stout and a Monk by the neck. I will once again retreat to my personal quarters for a short period of time. I will then be seen rejoining my house guests bearing the refreshment on a tray.'

'And would there be any charge for this?'

'None whatsoever. However, if you would wish to place an offering in the box by the door labelled "African Lepers", I could indicate a sum that would be appreciated by the Overseas Fathers in charge of those unfortunate dark souls.'

'Would that offering in any way approximate to the price of five pints of stout, a large Bush and a Monk by the neck?' I asked.

'To the penny,' was the reply.

Now I had seen everything.

'How long have you been operating like this?' I asked.

'Oh, about fifteen years.'

We stayed longer than we should have, got used to the system, sang a few bawdy songs accompanied by trombone mouthpiece and became overly familiar with a section of the clientele.

I told her I was in love with her.

'All the strangers say that,' was her coy reply.

We eventually stumbled out of the unpub and found our way back to the dance-hall, where we took to the stage and played loudly to fewer than a score of people who didn't want to hear us.

By midnight the place was packed . . . approximately fifteen-hundred people in various stages of decomposition.

There had been a festival of sorts in a nearby village that day and the task of handing out prizes to winners of the fancy-dress parade was entrusted to the band. I, being the talking head on stage, was allotted the chore.

Third prize went to the village idiot. He had a huge head dotted with bulbous growths, and an alarming habit of growling if anyone came to close.

His prize-winning fancy dress consisted solely of a placard draped about his neck upon which was scrawled: 'I'VE GOT A TIGER IN MY TANK'.

I called his name over the microphone and, from the back of the hall, he shuffled gamely towards the stage to receive his prize. *En route* he was subjected to enthusiastic slaps, hard punches and painful kicks from a joshing audience. Just a bit of encouragement, you see.

By the time he had reached my giving hand, he had been battered almost senseless and was in bad shape, bleeding unevenly and on the verge of losing whatever degree of consciousness he had started the night with.

He crawled towards me whimpering softly, and I gave him a small box of Black Magic chocolates which tumbled from his enfeebled hand.

Fearing he was badly injured, I called a bouncer, who

carried him backstage into what masqueraded as our dressing room, with a promise that he would receive some form of cursory medical examination.

I was slightly worried about him, and ten minutes later went backstage to see if he was OK, only to be informed that he had recovered and left.

He was last seen making his way down the road riding a bicycle.

Whistling, apparently.

Maybe he was going to Farrelly's not to buy a drink.

I wished I'd gone with him and not bought one either.

A 'CELEBRITY' AT THE
CROSSROADS

IT IS EARLY 1993 and I am ill at ease. The 'Troubles' have taken a downturn and I fear that a full-blown civil war can't be far away.

The people of Northern Ireland are irretrievably alienated. The world pities us, Britain is bored with our interminable quarrel and the Tory Government has all but given up. It's a dangerous time.

The mood on the streets is ugly, people hate each other as never before and the scum are organised.

Encouraged and nourished for twenty-five years, the hate appears to be coming to a head. A sophisticated hate, all-encompassing and a mystery to strangers. Something deep-down and medieval. I fear the cork may pop out of the bottle very soon, unleashing an evil that exists within many of our otherwise sane people. An evil that may manifest itself in a bloodbath.

We are, I am convinced, more than capable of it.

I have decided that I don't want to be there when it happens. This presents a problem because, career-wise, I've never had it so good.

I am at the helm of the most popular daily radio show in Northern Ireland and the host of a successful Friday-night television talk-show. As a profitable by-product, I spend happy hours opening sparkling supermarkets, slobbering over small babies, flattering young housewives and humouring old women, all the while smiling mechanically, enjoying the kind of regional fame that prompts people to giggle hysterically when they are introduced to me; asking stupid questions that they usually regret later, such as 'Aren't you taller?', to which I can only reply, 'No.'

I am a 'personality' in a country about to implode. I am comfortable working on Northern Ireland radio but feel like a prostitute on television and know in my heart that I am not prepared to undergo the humiliation and forfeiture of self-respect that is required to mount a serious assault on the light entertainment end of the medium.

Radio it has to be, then.

I look across the sea and consider England a possibility. Radio 2 appeals to me as a likely resting place but I fear I have created the wrong impression and will have to wait until someone who likes me is in charge.

I am too old for Radio 1, not interested in Radio 3, congenitally unfit for Radio 5, but am astonished to discover from general feedback that occasional monologues I have written and recorded for Radio 4 seem to have gone down quite well. This was the last thing I had expected. My initial impression of Radio 4 was that those who were most enthusiastic about it seemed to hold the opinion that intelligence must not be allowed to exist in the absence of an aggressive Oxbridge education worn thuggishly on the sleeve.

Maybe I was wrong.

Maybe there was another potential audience out there, one that was not particularly interested in the history of Pamela Anderson's tits or the alcoholism and failed whirlwind romances of people who appeared in *Coronation Street*, but, alternatively, an audience that couldn't stomach the Archers or James Naughtie either, and who listened grim-faced to Ned Sherrin, Ian Hislop, Alan Coren and other 'wits'.

Maybe there was room for something a little less smug.

It was a long shot, but one worth considering.

I visited London from time to time, and floated about Broadcasting House recording various little pieces for radio and talking to friends who worked there. I had been told by the more cynical among them that Radio 4 was a network under the jackboot of a small but vocal portion of the listening audience who were dedicated to preserving what remained of the ethos of Empire.

This hardcore audience was apparently reluctant to countenance change of any kind and clung desperately to the network as the last remnant of the Way Things Used to Be.

The common consensus on the inside was that many of the 'hardcore' audience felt let down by Government, Monarchy, Church and the Education System, tending to regard Radio 4 as the last defence against whatever mob of lager-guzzling, baseball-cap-wearing, glue-sniffing modern Visigoths or Vandals was supposedly hammering on the stout wooden doors of Broadcasting House. I wondered what it would be like to work there, knowing that the network attracted extremely talented people who beavered away behind the scenes as producers, researchers and ancillary dogsbodies.

So, if there were talented individuals working behind the scenes, how come so many of the people who presented and took part in many of the programmes sounded like pompous wankers?

It didn't make sense.

I would often discuss this in the George (BBC watering hole) with a friend of mine who worked on the inside . . . my Deep Throat.

'It doesn't make sense,' I would say.

He would sip his pint and sigh. 'That's what the listeners want; constant reassurance that the status quo remains unaltered. All we can do at the moment is wait until all the old China hands and Thatcher-soundalikes living in Eastbourne die off,' Deep Throat would say. 'People who work in Radio 4 are afraid of the audience. We're under siege.'

'Particularly under siege at the moment?' I asked.

'Not just now. All of the time. You just try tinkering with the Shipping Forecast and see what happens. They'd probably march on Downing Street. Look what happened when we moved *Woman's Hour* from afternoon to morning. A public outcry!'

'But you got away with that, didn't you?' I said.

'Only just. Frightened the life out of us.'

'What's wrong with these people? It's only radio,' I replied.

'That's where you're wrong. It's more than radio. What's wrong with these people is that they have nowhere else to go. If you or I don't like a programme on the radio, we switch to another station. These people regard it as a personal insult. If they don't like a programme, it's off with its head!'

He ordered more drink.

'Surely that's the way the system should work, though,' I said. 'If the majority of listeners don't like a programme, isn't it right that it should go?' I suggested.

'That's the whole point. They're not the majority at all. A small minority calls the shots . . . the storm troopers of Middle England.'

'And what about the rest of the punters?' I asked.

'Have you ever written to the *Daily Telegraph* or the ex-*Thunderer* about a radio programme you didn't like?'

'No,' I replied.

'Do you know of anyone who has?'

'No.'

'Well, we're talking here about the kind of people who want to bring back the birch and castrate homosexuals. They know best.'

I was no stranger to this line of thought. I was from Northern Ireland and, therefore, knew all about rabid intolerance.

I felt sorry for him as I watched him drain his pint.

This was getting to him.

'But who exactly are these people?' I asked.

'Fucked if I know,' he said. 'They're like the National Guard, more like Crusaders, actually, and they're constantly sniffing the air for signs of change. Our hands are tied.'

I could see his point.

'But Radio 4 isn't all that bad,' I said. 'I like some of it, Nick

Ross, for instance, and sometimes Melvyn Bragg's not too annoying.'

'They're more or less exceptions to the rule. Yes, you're right. And Alistair Cooke's not bad either.'

I said nothing. I had met Alistair Cooke before, and a crotchety old bastard he was too.

Our paths had crossed in New York, at the BBC studios in Rockefeller Plaza, where a couple of colleagues and I were putting together a St Patrick's Day programme for Radio Ulster. We had a looming deadline with a satellite dish and were under considerable pressure.

Whilst we were working feverishly at editing machines, a female minion popped her head round the door.

'Mr Cooke's coming,' she announced.

She looked nervous but we paid her no particular attention.

'I said Mr Cooke's coming,' she repeated.

'So?' one of us said.

'You'll have to leave immediately,' she added tersely.

'Where does he record his programme?' I asked.

'Next door,' she replied.

'That's OK, then,' I said. 'We won't be interfering with him in any way.'

'He won't allow it,' she answered.

'Why?'

'Because he'll know you're here.'

'What difference does it make to him if we're here or not? He won't see us or hear us. We have a deadline to meet.'

'He has to walk through here to get to the studio next door. He'll see you. He won't like it,' she said.

'Fuck him. We don't mind if we see *him*. Why should he be bothered about seeing us?'

'You'll have to leave.'

Before I could answer, the great Alistair Cooke walked in and looked at us as if we were plague rats. He did not address us directly. 'Who are these people?' he demanded imperiously of the minion.

She mumbled something about St Patrick's Day that made

little impression upon him.

'Get them out of here. They're in my eye line!' he announced, and swept into the studio next door.

I couldn't help thinking that if he'd been a younger man talking to us like that he would have had to contend with something else in his eye line that more resembled a balled fist. However, not wishing to reciprocate unpleasantness, we meekly filed out and hung about in the corridor for an hour until he'd finished recording his *Letter from America*, anxiously watching the precious minutes slip away.

He eventually tottered out, ignored us completely and stalked off.

'We need to broaden the listenership,' continued Deep Throat. 'There are people all over the country who would like to listen to Radio 4 but usually feel like putting a boot through the radio whenever they do accidentally lend an ear to it. There have to be people out there who can't hack Dave Lee Travis or Jimmy Young. Has our education system failed us entirely? There must be people out there who want to hear interesting programmes presented by people who don't make them want to puke. At the moment Radio 4 is local radio for Middle England. It's supposed to be a national network, for fuck's sake! It has little to offer averagely intelligent, sane people who live elsewhere. The real people.'

Deep Throat was getting excited. I worried about him. I had spent all my life with the real people and was concerned about his optimism.

'Well, are there any plans to do something about this?' I asked.

'Maybe,' said Deep Throat. 'The suits are thinking about it upstairs.'

Good for the suits. Maybe he was right. To the averagely intelligent, well-adjusted listener, much of the content of Radio 4 programmes possibly did sound like the kind of university common-room bollocks that is only appreciated within a closed circle.

If one assumes that the purpose of a university education is to enable the student to recognise the sound of people talking bollocks when he hears it, then one must necessarily conclude that this has yet to occur to many of those presenting and participating in a distressingly large number of these radio programmes.

So, a heady mix of the good and the unspeakable.

As Deep Throat turned to someone else and eagerly repeated what he had just told me, I left the George with much to think about.

This was scary territory.

Nevertheless, it was better than staying at home.

Maybe I could find a little programme somewhere on Radio 4 where I wouldn't frighten the horses. After all, I had been received quite well so far, and there was no reason why that should not continue to be the case.

I decided on a little reconnaissance and, to this end, sought out a producer friend of mine.

I had always liked him. He was affable, relaxed and informed.

'How would a fellow go about getting himself a little weekly programme on Radio 4 that wouldn't be too great a burden to bear?' I asked.

'Like what?' he replied.

'Something not too difficult. Something that would allow a man to spend three or four days a week in London. Something that would buy him time to have a good look around?'

He sucked on his pipe. 'Fancy a permanent move then?'

'Eventually. If God is good.'

'Why do you want to work over here?' he asked.

'To avoid ethnic cleansing,' I answered.

'I'll ask around,' he replied.

He seemed to understand.

I was content to let the hare sit.

Let's see what happens.

Anyway, this was not my immediate concern. I had some travelling to do.

WHITE MICE AND MAPLE
SYRUP

SOMEWHERE IN THE middle of Amsterdam, I find myself sitting bolt upright on a sofa belonging to an apartment inhabited by people whom I do not know.

My mouth tastes like an Arab's underpants and my ears are assailed by the sound of a wailing human voice belonging to a chinless Australian wearing a herring-bone overcoat. He is accompanying himself on an eighteenth-century pipe-organ that fills half the room.

The windows and fittings rattle frighteningly as he approaches the climax of a song that I chillingly recognise as 'There's No Business Like Showbusiness'.

I am disturbed to discover that an alarmingly large number of white mice scurry dizzily and untrammelled across the floor, watched dully by an equally white husky dog with pricked-up ears.

A slim, swarthy youth leans on a corner of the great organ, tapping his foot to the pulse of the music and staring disturbingly in my direction. His unseasonal headgear, long leather boots and riding crop confirm the information I receive later that he is a Turkish rent-boy from the upmarket riding stables next door.

The purpose of his presence is unclear.

Asleep at the other end of the sofa is a long-haired, angel-faced young man with a pale complexion. He's a suicidal Norwegian disc jockey who has come to Amsterdam to kill himself. When working, he broadcasts a daily record request show from within the Arctic Circle. When the long night falls, as it regularly does at six-monthly intervals, he becomes severely depressed and frequently flings himself into a nearby lake, from which he is routinely dragged out alive by good friends who know to keep an eye on him. He is hoping for better luck here in a more liberal environment where drowning in peace should be easier.

There seems to be some mildly illegal action taking place in an adjoining room, out of which staggers a scantily clad young woman who has earlier described herself to me as an orphaned junkie.

She flings her head recklessly in the direction of an open log fire. When her rat-tailed cranium emerges unscathed, I am relieved to discover that this apparent disregard for naked flame is merely an efficient means of igniting the large spliff which now dangles loosely from her blotched lips.

As she returns slowly to her room, I see through the doorway what appears to be a burly man of perhaps Ethiopian origin, wearing some form of feathered ceremonial head-dress. He is at ease with himself.

The music ceases and the chinless organist rushes suddenly to the open window, out of which he screams obscenities at passers-by in the street two floors below.

He then tugs lovingly at a cable that snakes ominously from a socket on the wall down to the street via the window. The cable is attached to a parked Mercedes sedan, rendering the vehicle electrically live and dangerous, if not fatal, to the touch.

This is the idea, of course . . . to deter thieves and unwanted grubby handprints on the vehicle's smooth, white finish. I regard this as being a shade draconian but the yelling, singing, blaspheming owner of the vehicle has no such qualms.

He returns to the organ and resumes his recital by poking out the opening notes of 'Guantanamera'.

As the tune proceeds, the decibel level in the room rises dramatically, causing a metallic boomerang to dislodge itself from the wall and clang noisily on to the wooden floor, from which it is immediately expertly snapped by the slavering jaws of the white husky, which then scampers from the room, slithering on the polished wooden floor, scattering white mice in its wake. Thin pink legs desperately paw the empty air.

It is Queen's Day in Amsterdam, a public holiday during which the inhabitants sell all their unwanted household goods in the street whilst getting drunk and making much noise. It's the biggest car-boot sale in the world.

The brown cafés are doing excellent business and my companion and I have spent way too much time in one of them. We are in a trance-like state and close to the edge. Furthermore, we have foolhardily accepted an invitation to a party in this apartment and I am growing increasingly nervous. Sociologically interesting though this gathering may be, this is not why we are here.

We are in Amsterdam on behalf of the BBC as part of a tour of five European capital cities to record material for radio documentaries of which an integral part is an investigation into the sudden proliferation of Irish pubs in Berlin, Amsterdam, Paris, Rome and Barcelona.

Suddenly, being Irish is chic. Irish people aren't used to being liked, never mind thought fashionable, so this is a considerable burden to place on a race that is accustomed to being tolerated at best, and at worst ignored and pitied, if not downright despised.

I am here to witness the Greening of the Continent. During the course of the last four years, twelve hundred Irish pubs have opened in Europe and Greater Asia.

I am here to discover why.

We have already visited Berlin and encountered our first European Irish pub there.

The Berlin Wall had been dismantled fairly recently, and at the Brandenburg Gate, shifty nomadic types were flogging Red Army paraphernalia to plump tourists.

I reluctantly resisted the shady offer of a Red Army

general's braided peaked cap and deflected the seller by telling him that I was from Ulster and knew friends who might be interested in a fully functioning armed MiG 15 fighter plane at the right price . . . just the thing to smarten up the squaddies in South Armagh.

His feet pawed the ground awkwardly like a horse and he mumbled something in a Central European tongue. I reassured him by laughing the hearty laugh of the innocent and crossing his palm with too many Deutschmarks in exchange for a small lump of rock in a plastic bag that may or may not have been a piece of the late Berlin Wall.

Bearing the questionably historic masonry, I marched into East Berlin Proper and negotiated a wide, ruined street. I had scribbled an address on a piece of paper and was assured that I was heading in the right direction. There was an Irish pub down there . . . somewhere.

As I walked and took in my surroundings, I had a vague sense of *déjà vu*. It was the East Berliners, the people on the street. I had seen them before . . . somewhere.

The West Berlin I had just left was full of Real Germans; pink-faced, stern, neat, law-abiding, thoroughly dislikeable but remarkably organised as they went about the business of doing everything better than anybody else in the world.

East Berlin was different. I was prepared for a dishevelled city but unprepared for the people.

Pale-faced, unwell-looking men stood at street corners sucking dog-ends and flapping their arms to keep warm as they all talked at the same time. Uniformly dressed in standard Oxfam garb, they averted their gaze as I passed. Their self-esteem seemed nil and a great deal of their time was spent coming to the aid of motorists driving ugly Trabant cars constructed of stiffened cardboard; cars that required a communal push when they regularly and unaccountably spluttered to a halt at major road junctions and other inconvenient locations.

These were spent men. Men with no hope.

The women seemed generally more active, as women

usually are when men aren't in control. Dowdy women with bad complexions and stout, blue-veined legs, shabbily dressed and walking with arms folded, trailing snot-blest, awkward, ill-fed children who weren't dressed for the weather.

In a moment of great clarity I realised that I had grown up with people just like these. They were East Germans, of course, but they looked as if they had lived in Northern Ireland all their lives.

These were my people.

I understood.

We were one.

I marvelled at the spectacular incompetence of the Russians. It takes a remarkable talent to destroy the spirit and the economy of a country full of Germans.

But what would these people want with an Irish pub?

They may have looked Irish but presumably that was where it ended.

Didn't they have enough misery and drudgery in their own lives without importing more people who acted and looked like them from a green land far away that had been bombed by their Luftwaffe parents?

What use would they find for a pub that boasted a clutch of granite-jawed traditional musicians clustered in a corner, sawing away on dun-coloured fiddles at a never-ending tune that sounded like the one before and frowning sternly at patrons who talked during the tin-whistle solos?

What would they want with overpriced pints of muddy, imported Guinness when they had perfectly good bierkellers of their own to carouse and shout German oaths in?

Who amongst them would want to sit on a bar stool and feel obliged to relate their life story to a man with a full head of hair and a smelly shirt, whose sole purpose in life was the cadging of free drink?

Who wanted to hear about the Armed Struggle in Ulster when he'd had the Stasie breathing down his neck since Hitler took the dive, or be told about narrow escapes from bomb blasts in Belfast when his own city had been flattened to

Hiroshima levels by the combined bombing might of the largest fleet of aircraft ever pitted against any one nation at any given time in the history of mankind?

Beats me . . .

I sensed I was nearing my destination and, scanning the bleak terrain, noticed a curious building occupying an otherwise derelict corner of a bullet-holed, cobbled street.

It looked like a pub, but I must confess that I was thrown by the sight of the tail of a light aircraft protruding from its gable wall.

Strange people gathered at the entrance.

One of them, a tall woman wearing sparse, spangled clothing that revealed a wide expanse of naked midriff, approached and muttered something Teutonic in an unnaturally deep voice. Her heavy facial make-up failed to conceal a generous growth of stubble on her chin and a cursory examination of her exposed, hairy biceps led me to take evasive action. I was not in the mood for a man in my life at that moment.

I stepped inside what was indeed a pub. The place looked as if it had been designed by a crazed pilot.

It was sparsely populated. Most of the action was taking place outside on the street. The bar-top and surrounding furnishings seemed to be made of jagged sheet metal. Disembodied ejector seats from fighter planes hung suspended from the ceiling, as did a number of slowly circling propellers. On closer examination of the bar-top, I found that it was fashioned from the wing of some small flying craft. All the pub's fixtures and fittings were discarded aeroplane parts.

The place was aerodynamically sound.

I sat myself down on a piece of fuselage and was approached by a gum-chewing waitress who looked refreshingly normal.

I ordered a Heineken.

The waitress hesitated for a moment and returned five minutes later with, to my surprise, a small roasted chicken.

I pointed in wonder at the scorched carcass.

'Beer?' I asked.

'*Hähnchen,*' she replied.

Ah . . . I see . . . linguistic confusion. Similar pronunciation, different meanings.

I resignedly accepted the steaming poultry and did what I should have done in the first place. I ordered a beer.

She brought me a bottle of Heineken.

I shouldn't have been surprised. My German was minimal. I had visited a supermarket earlier that morning to buy some toilet items and later brushed my teeth with fish paste. I hesitate to recommend this.

Gnawing at the *Hähnchen* and sipping the Heineken, I noticed a solitary man sitting at the bar staring at me. He rose, smiled, walked towards my aluminium table and sat down on an adjacent piece of shrapnel. 'You're from home, aren't you?' he said.

'Isn't everybody?' I replied.

His face darkened somewhat. I was sorry I had been flippant.

'Irish?' I asked.

'Yeah. You too, by the look of ya,' he said. 'Enjoying your meal?'

'It's delicious. I wish I'd ordered it.'

'Wha?'

'Never mind,' says I.

He was personable enough, dressed in regulation Irishman-away-from-home crumpled jumper and soiled jeans. We talked a lot of Irish talk, preliminary sparring bluster. It was established that he was from Dublin, I from the North, and wouldn't Ireland be a grand little country if we all learned to get along with each other and respect the different points of view of others who were, after all, in their own way, just as Irish as the rest of us. The usual bollocks.

He took care to establish that I was from what people in Ireland refer to as a 'Nationalist' background, and when I asked him what the fuck he was doing in East Berlin, he scanned the room and leaned forwards to within two inches of my face.

'I'm on the run,' he whispered.

'Political?' I enquired mildly.

He nodded.

'What are you wanted for?' I asked gently.

'Dis 'n' dat,' he replied. 'And a bit o' the other.'

I began to feel uneasy. I could live with dis and dat but had never been a man comfortable with the other.

I rapidly changed the subject.

'There's an Irish pub somewhere on this street, isn't there?' I said amiably. 'Wouldn't that be where you should hang out?'

He spat, causing the waitress to cock an ear at the unfamiliar sound of a gob of Hibernian mucus striking her pristine floor.

'Jasus, no! Not for me. I wouldn't drink there. Full of poofters and little shites with mobile phones. Wearing baseball caps turned the wrong way round.'

'Show me where it is then,' I suggested. 'I'll buy you a pint. You don't have to stay there if you don't want to.'

'Right,' says he, and off we went.

On the way out I asked him if this strange aerial watering-hole had a name.

'It's called the Black Box,' he replied.

Of course.

We shuffled down the street until we came upon the inevitable green façade. I peered through the stained-glass front door adorned with a shamrock and prised it open just enough to take in the ambience.

The interior was a coffin of mahogany, the décor so familiar that I half-expected to see my Uncle Jimmy standing at the bar telling lies about greyhounds, or indeed my Uncle Amby (short for Ambrose) who was always with him. Fate had dealt Uncle Amby a cruel blow. Life was always going to be difficult for a one-armed man named Amby.

But I digress.

A man with uncontrollable ginger hair swayed in a corner,

flailing an acoustic guitar whilst bravely warbling 'The Stone Outside Dan Murphy's Door'.

I saw limp chips being consumed absent-mindedly by limp men. An open fire stuffed with artificial peat roared merrily. Pictures of icons adorned the wall. The complete range, from Michael Collins to Dana. Solitary men stared gloomily into their pints, presumably thinking of Ireland. I sensed the usual air of traditional hopelessness.

And yes, gathered in another corner was the new generation, those who had grasped the Celtic Tiger by the tail, mostly poofters who mingled freely with the little shites who had mobile phones. They were wearing baseball caps turned the wrong way round.

I turned to face my shadowy new-found friend. 'Fuck this. Let's go back to the Black Box.'

I was fully aware of the irony. I was spurning what should be dear to me and willingly walking the mean, bullet-pocked streets of East Berlin towards a group of German transvestites in the company of a fugitive from the British Government who was prepared to fight and die for Ireland provided Ireland did not expect him to like Irish people.

I later observed him stepping into a taxi with a man who was dressed in an off-the-shoulder diamanté-studded evening dress. My mind drifts.

I am jerked awake by sudden pain in the region of my left shoulder. It is being pounded by the fist of a suicidal Norwegian disc jockey.

'He vants you to sing!'

'Who does?' I stutter, maddened by fatigue.

The terminal DJ jabs a finger in the direction of the man at the controls of the pipe-organ, whose hands are poised at the keyboard. The organist smiles broadly, revealing hideous teeth.

'Sing the song you sing zis afternoon. Ve loved it so,' urges the suddenly cheerful Scandinavian.

The great organ trumpets a deafening B flat major chord. I feel the beady eyes of white mice upon me.

A Turkish rent-boy waits expectantly. An Ethiopian has passed out on the hearth. An orphaned junkie is enveloped in smoke. A husky pants.

Now I remember.

To thunderous notes from the extended pipes of the mighty instrument, I open a parched throat, from which come the unmistakable opening lines of . . .

'Come back, Paddy Reilly, to Bally . . . james . . . duff . . .'

LATER THAT YEAR

It is the day after Hallowe'en and I am in Los Angeles sitting in the lobby of a Santa Monica hotel being watched carefully by the hotel manager. I have heard disturbing news from home.

On Hallowe'en night, men wearing balaclavas walked into a Stroke City bar that I know well and shouted 'Trick or treat!' Apparently, the drinkers laughed at what appeared a harmless though tasteless seasonal jape. The laughter ceased abruptly when the intruders produced automatic weapons and generally opened fire. Many were killed or wounded. I could have been there. Had I not been here.

I am in Los Angeles to attend a glittering showbusiness fundraiser for the deserving poor and the oppressed of Ireland. I am to interview Hollywood stars. I should be excited, but I'm not.

Forty-eight hours ago I was standing in a function room of the Beverley Hills Hotel waiting for movie stars to be brought to me by an American fixer. Our hired American camera crew are relaxing between takes. The soundman is bronzed and sports a long ponytail. He is impossibly handsome and I tell him that if he lived in Ireland he could become a star just by showing up. He laughs and fishes a movie script from his inside pocket, urging me to read it. He tells me that he wrote it himself. Maybe I know somebody who would be interested?

I pass.

That's the way it is here. Everybody's a star who hasn't been discovered yet.

I had dined in a showbiz Hollywood restaurant the night before, where starlets come to be seen by the dining movie moguls. They stand by the bar (they never sit) and make frequent trips through the dining area to the ladies' powder room. The object of these journeys is to be seen walking across the floor. Stuff is strutted.

Every once in a while, one of these girls is beckoned by a movie fatcat and calling cards are exchanged. A direct hit is scored. It's demeaning and I love it.

I talk to a waiter who tells me that he is an actor between jobs. I humour him by saying that I think I recognise him.

He brightens and suggests that I may have seen him on television.

I pretend to rack my brains and, giving up, ask him what he has appeared in.

He tells me proudly that he was the psychopath who was killed in *Knot's Landing*.

Of course.

Our schedule is tight and we have a limited amount of time to catch the stars before they eat. I have already interviewed Angie Dickinson, John Wayne's son and a Disney. We are running out of time and Bob Hope is late. I am due to interview him between 8.30 and 8.45. It is now almost nine o'clock. Almost too late.

I turn to my producer, who seems unconcerned. 'Where the fuck's Bob Hope?'

'What did you say?'

'I said, where the fuck's Bob Hope? He was supposed to be here at eight thirty.'

My producer looks at me sympathetically and sighs. 'Remember what you have just said and dwell upon it. Who was your childhood comedy hero in the movies? Which Hollywood star would you have given anything to meet but knew that such a meeting was beyond your wildest dreams? Who? I want you to say his name. We talked about him on the plane coming over. Who was it?'

I pause.

'What was his name?' insists the producer.

'Um . . . Bob Hope.'

'Precisely,' he says. 'Have a little respect.'

'Well, where the fuck is he then?'

America always brings out the worst in me. I always get into trouble there. I never know what form it's going to take but know only that it is inevitable.

This time around, the trouble started innocently enough. I was occupying a modest room in the Santa Monica hotel and my producer had the room next door. We were just about to check out when I decided to have a shower. My friend said that he would go down to the lobby and settle the bill.

I emerged from the shower refreshed and in the fullness of time found myself dressed and ready to leave. Just one last phone call to make.

I lifted the receiver and dialled 9 for an outside extension. I had no success. I rang reception.

'Hello,' I said. 'This is me in Room 1328. May I have an outside line, please?'

There was a silence at the other end.

'Helloooo, may I have an outside line, please?' I repeated.

A reply came. 'I'm sorry, sir. Your room has been vacated, sir.'

'Pardon?' I said. 'Vacated?'

'Who are you, sir?' the voice asked.

'It's me, Mr Anderson in Room 1328. I've been here for three days.'

'I'm sorry, sir. You've checked out, sir.'

'But I'm still here, in my room. I'm still here.'

'No you're not, sir. You've checked out, sir.'

'But I am here,' I said. 'This is me speaking. I'm pretty certain that I am standing here at this moment speaking to you from my room in which I have spent the better part of three days. This is me. I know me. There can be no mistake.'

I began to understand. My friend had paid the bill. He had discharged my contractual obligations towards the hotel. They were no longer interested in me. I didn't exist. It's the corporate way. I was in no mood for this.

I continued. 'There's a perfectly logical explanation for this. I understand and appreciate fully that my friend has probably paid the bill. But I'm still here and would like to make a phone call from my room, for which I will pay when I emerge from what you call the elevator, which, as you can probably see, is directly opposite the reception desk from which I assume you are speaking to me right now. I cannot escape unless I throw myself out of the window. *Comprende?*'

I heard the clunk of a phone being urgently placed on a solid surface. I held on for thirty seconds. Another voice came on the line.

'Hi! Good morning, sir. My name is Ray Gould. I'm your hotel manager. I believe there is a problem. How may I resolve it?'

I explained the situation carefully, confident that common sense would prevail. He was, after all, a senior management figure.

'I'm sorry,' he replied. 'You can't make any calls. You've checked out, sir.'

I thought for a moment and, considering my response carefully, replied, 'Well, fuck you and your poxy hotel!'

I hung up and took the lift to the ground floor where breakfast awaited.

Stepping nimbly out, I glanced towards the reception desk where two men eyed me suspiciously as I made my way to a payphone in the lobby. I went about the mechanics of making a call. When my business was completed, I replaced the receiver and noticed immediately that there were now three men staring at me from the reception desk. I muttered the word 'house-dick' under my breath. It was a word I had never used before. It came straight out of my head from Hollywood. I realised that I was now getting into the spirit of things.

I joined my friend at the breakfast bar, and upon being told by the waitress to have a nice day, I enjoyed a hearty breakfast of eggs over easy, hash browns, charred bacon and squiggly things. Having some time to kill, we remained at the table, quietly reading newspapers comprised of many sections. Eventually I began to feel peckish again and examined the menu. The words 'Pancakes with Maple Syrup' caught my eye.

I again called the waitress, an attractive girl with impossibly white teeth, all thirty-two on public display, bared in a smile that would have put any seasoned air hostess to shame.

'How many pancakes covered in maple syrup would a man get if he ordered pancakes and maple syrup?' I enquired.

'A normal portion would be three pancakes, sir,' she replied slowly and carefully. Like something feral, she had sensed my mood.

'Well, how about this?' I said. 'As you are well aware, I've already had breakfast but find I need a little top-up. Now I don't think I could handle all three pancakes, so why don't you bring me one pancake covered in maple syrup and charge me for the full portion, of course.'

She bit her lip nervously and seemed to undergo some fierce internal struggle. 'Why . . . why don't I bring you the normal portion and you can eat one and leave the other two?' she suggested.

Here we go.

'Well, there are a number of reasons why I would prefer you didn't do that. Firstly, it's a waste of two perfectly edible pancakes covered with maple syrup for no valid reason; secondly, there are children starving all over the world; and thirdly, I've seen these pancakes before and I know that they're HUGE MOTHERFUCKERS and if I see three heaped on a plate I won't want any of them, whereas if I see only one pancake, I will want to eat it. It's a thing I have about pancakes, a psychological thing. Do you have a problem with that?'

I sensed she was beginning to panic. Maybe it was because

she had never before heard the words 'psychological' and 'pancake' used in the same sentence. Come to think of it, neither had I.

She looked at me as if I were a rabid dog. She spoke. 'Let me just check, sir.'

She disappeared behind some walnut panelling and returned presently, accompanied by a smartly dressed individual who walked like a man wearing someone else's shoes. He reminded me of a meerkat, not only because of his erect, rigid posture, but also because he sniffed the air as he strode along.

He stopped at our table and clasped his hands behind his back. I knew who he was.

'Hi! My name is Ray Gould. I'm the hotel manager. Another problem, Mr Anderson?'

'Now do you believe I'm here?' I countered.

'Hotel policy, sir. Are we experiencing some difficulty?'

'Yes,' I replied. 'I'm afraid we are. I want one pancake and I'm willing to pay for three of the fuckers but she says I have to take three and not eat two of them but I don't want three because if I get three I won't want any of them and she doesn't seem capable of grasping the fact that there are people in this world like me who are easily put off things . . . like pancakes.' My voice trailed away. I realised that I was being unreasonable but it was too late to stop now.

He waved the waitress away, glanced uneasily at the other diners, and moved a little closer to my face. 'We have procedures and ways of doing things here. I regret to inform you that we are unable to comply with your request at this juncture. And I would ask you to modify your language. We have other guests.'

By this time pancakes were the furthest thing from my mind. This was a guy thing.

The devil took hold of me and I decided to employ the ultimate weapon. Looking the hotel manager straight in the eye, I reached into my pocket, produced a packet of cigarettes and withdrew one of those deadly white cylinders that I knew

Americans hated more than almost anything else in the world.

This action had the desired effect. His eyes widened and his mouth opened slowly in horror. I grinned evilly as I put the cigarette to my lips.

'I must inform you that it is against Californian law to smoke in a restaurant, sir! I have to warn you that you are committing an offence and I am, therefore, perfectly within my rights to call the police, which I shall not hesitate to do!'

I knew he could call the police. I had heard of this sort of thing before. I had somehow sensed that he was a Cigarette Nazi, and I was right.

The unlit cigarette dangled loosely from my lips.

I felt like a gunslinger.

Something was happening to me. I was gripped by a sudden, reckless madness and, to my surprise, found myself speaking in a slow, Southern Texas drawl.

'Gonna call the cigarette cops, huh? Ain't no crime till I light the crittur.'

I had become John Wayne.

It was a Mexican stand-off. Snatches of Hollywood dialogue raced across my brain.

Fill your hand, you sonuvabitch!

Eat dirt, sodbuster!

I deal in lead!

My thumb was poised over my GI Zippo petroleum lighter. The weapon was cocked. There was one in the breech. Just one squeeze and it was all over.

The voice of common sense screamed in my brain. Was I prepared to break the law simply because I was invisible in a hotel and couldn't order a single pancake? I knew what these people were like.

The hotel manager hated me. I could tell. He would call the police and God knows what he would tell them. It was his word against mine. He would make me pay dearly for daring to be different in corporate America.

I could feel the eyes of the other diners boring into the back of my head. My heart beat wildly and the Zippo lighter went in and out of focus before my smarting eyes. A bead of sweat trickled down my forehead. I could see my colleague's lips move but I couldn't hear what I knew in my heart were his desperate pleas urging me to see sense and abort this foolish course of action.

The air-conditioner hummed quietly and a score of people held their breath.

I had made my decision.

In the interests of freedom of choice, my thumb fell, a blue flame shot into the air and ignited the business end of a Marlboro Light. Acrid fumes polluted the filtered air.

What happened next was a blur. The hotel manager squealed with rage and rushed headlong towards a phone. My colleague grabbed me by the shirt collar and we suddenly found ourselves running for our lives through the desirable beachfront properties of Santa Monica. Fugitives from the law . . . Butch and Sundance.

Of course, we had to return for our luggage.

We blamed the heat.

They were easy on us.

Never did like pancakes, anyway.

'ANDERSON COUNTRY'

SCANNING THE *Los Angeles Times* in Las Vegas airport on the eve of my return home, I saw that the Shankill Road in Belfast had been bombed. More innocent men, women and children had died for nothing.

The screw was tightening. All-out cleansing was near.

Returning to Northern Ireland through a murky sky during the small hours of a frosty Monday morning, I left the plane and trudged listlessly through the dreariness that was Belfast International Airport, glancing at the pinched, grey face of a stunted man who was sweeping out the deserted lounge. He caught my eye and leaning lightly on the shaft of his brush, fixed me with a glance. 'Bit of a tan, eh?' he said conspiratorially from the corner of his mouth, the way some Belfast people do.

'Yeah, I suppose I have, a bit,' I answered automatically.

'Anywhere nice?' he continued.

'Ah . . . Los Angeles, Vegas.'

'It's a wonder you wouldn't have had a bit of sense and stayed there when you had half a chance.'

Not this time, I thought. But somewhere else, soon.

'Enjoy your trip?' said the educated English voice on the other end of the line.

It was a producer with whom I had worked on Radio 4.

'Not as many fleshpots as I would have liked,' I replied.

'Something's come up that might be of interest to you,' he said.

'Yeah?'

'Yes, they're trying out people for a new daily afternoon show on Radio 4. Looking for somebody to present it who's not too stupid. Somebody with the common touch but who won't alarm the listeners. Gonna do regional stories of interest, phone calls and regular stuff, sort of Radio 2 with a brain. Interested?'

'That's a bit of a departure,' I said.

'Isn't it just? Word is they're really going to push this thing. It might be good to get on board early. There's bound to be flak when it gets off the ground, though.'

'Jesus,' I said. 'That's the last thing I want. I've had enough flak, thank you. And what is it? Five days a week? That's a grind. I want less work, not more. Who are they looking at?'

'Four or five people will be tried out shortly.'

'Who?'

'Usual suspects. You should have a crack at it. What have you got to lose?'

Everything, I thought. Probably be eaten alive.

I said so.

'No, the time is right.'

'What happens if it goes belly-up?' I asked.

'If it goes belly-up, it'll go belly-up big. If it works, it'll work big. There'll be no in-betweens here.'

'Let me think about it.' I hung up the phone.

It was a gamble, but why not go for it? I'd never get the job in a million years, so what harm would be done by taking a crack at it? Besides, I had never auditioned before. It might be fun. Anyway, who dares, wins.

Phone calls were exchanged and I found myself once more in the foyer of Broadcasting House, waiting for the summons to record a 'pilot' programme. Other potential presenters would do the same and, after results were held up to the light and entrails examined, the Chosen One would be announced . . . Darwinian but fair.

I sat happily watching the broadcasting world flutter by. Robert Robinson sailed past trailing pipe-smoke and wearing an enormous floppy hat. I made a mental note to never, ever wear similar headgear. There's something about a man wearing an extravagant, wide-brimmed hat that invites the world to hit him.

A wan Anthea Turner sat in a huddle with glum, spotty teenagers, showing little sign that she would soon become what I believe is now known as a Babe.

Steve Wright walked morosely by, his long, sad face at odds with the cheeky-chappie, happening, jolly disc jockey that millions knew and loved.

There was an air of briskness about the place that you don't usually find in Ireland. As a race, we are relatively brisk-free. I wondered if I might find this a handicap. Everybody, except Steve Wright, seemed happy, efficient and on top of whatever the world might throw at them.

I had never felt that way.

I was ushered upstairs and introduced to a group of young, bright, cheery people whom I instantly liked.

Modus operandi explained, I was shown into a hermetically sealed office with briefing notes on people I was about to interview, and invited to write a script.

I caused some alarm by asking for a pen and paper. It was suggested that I use a computer, and a short silence ensued when I explained that I didn't know how. A pen was swiftly found. I duly swotted potted notes about a retired Russian spy and other odd characters I was to interview. Armed with linking script, germs of arguments and suggested questions, I was brought to the studio to perform.

Convinced I had little chance of being offered the job, I decided to have a bit of fun and swashbuckled my way through the pilot, alarming only the retired Russian spy who took exception to what he described as my 'insouciant manner'. After all, this was no laughing matter.

It was to me.

The programme ended and I was surprised to find that

those around me had mistakenly interpreted my 'insouciance' as evidence of 'a man in control'.

I was about to open my mouth to refute this when something stopped me. Let them think that if they like, I thought. It's a free country. I returned home and, as expected, heard nothing.

A couple of weeks later I received a call from one of the producers. 'We want you to do another one,' he said.

'Another what?' I replied.

'Another pilot.'

'Why?'

'They want to check out your journalistic bite.'

'I don't have journalistic bite. I'm allergic to it,' I replied. 'I'm not a journalist. I've met journalists. I don't want to be one.'

'They want to see if you can handle weighty interviews.'

'Tell them I can't. And tell them this. I don't want to. I get into enough trouble over here by being light.'

'They insist. I think they like you. You're in with a good chance. You wouldn't have been called back otherwise.'

'But I don't want to do any serious stuff. This new daily programme isn't supposed to be about that, is it? If you want a weighty, worthy interviewer go upstairs to the BBC canteen and throw a stone in any direction. You're bound to hit one. There's two to every table.'

'Do it anyway. What have you got to lose?'

There it was again. The question was dogging me.

I relented and submitted to another pilot.

This time I was to chair a quasi-political discussion, something so boring that I can't even remember what it was about. I made what I thought were the expected noises, hated every second of it, and almost fell asleep. I had never come to terms with the enjoyment many people derive from political debates, probably because most people's political views are fashioned from their sense of having a stake in their own society . . . an unshakeable belief that their views mattered and would always be taken into consideration.

I was from a different school. Living in Northern Ireland during my formative years and seeing, from the hard end, a rotten-to-the-core democracy that didn't work, I knew beyond doubt that it didn't matter what I thought.

What mattered was what the Other Bastards thought.

I was congenitally dysfunctional, incapable of caring, and a risk to civilised, reasoned debate . . . a lost cause. Maybe I could be cured in time and eventually behave like a solid, useful citizen, but I was not prepared to hold my breath waiting for this to happen.

When the pilot was over, I thought, that's it. Ah well, it was worth coming to London, if only to see a few good movies, browse in second-hand bookshops, look at girls walking down Oxford Street, and stare happily at grumpy Radio 1 disc jockeys.

I went home and was informed almost immediately that I had been selected as the presenter of Radio 4's new flagship daily afternoon programme, as yet untitled.

The nightmare had begun.

It was fine to begin with. I installed myself in a well-appointed, centrally located bijou flat just off Marylebone High Street and looked forward to the task at hand.

I decided to stop smoking and ate therapeutic grapes.

The programme was titled *Anderson Country* and the operation took over the entire seventh floor of Broadcasting House. A huge staff was assembled and meetings proliferated like rabbits. I attended some of these meetings but spoke little. Everybody seemed to know what they were doing and there seemed little need for my input. What did I know?

Anyway, I was a little overawed by the scale of the enterprise. I had been a one-man band as far as radio was concerned and, on reflection, my chief gripe about television was the sheer number of people needed to man the ship. I had always felt uncomfortable taking other people's views into consideration as I habitually worked on instinct. If it feels right, do it. A visceral thing.

Problems always arose when I had to explain why I wanted to do things in a certain way. It wasn't enough to cite 'gut feeling' when others produced complicated reasons why things should be done differently.

Consequently, due to my lack of enthusiasm for heated debate, I usually gave in and did what the majority wanted . . . the easy option. Always a mistake.

I was genetically incapable of being a team player.

I didn't worry about this on *Anderson Country*. The producers, research staff and dogsbodies were all extremely capable. They were the cream of their craft. I was very happy to let them get on with it. I was happy to be the Talking Head. Anyway, the brief was straightforward. *Anderson Country* was designed to exhibit the human face of Radio 4.

I was all for it.

'Ordinary' people would be encouraged to appear on the programme to talk about what concerned them, good regional stories would be given more air time and dealt with in depth, subjects with a broad appeal would be tackled in an intelligent manner and the relevant people would be wheeled in to contribute their tuppenceworth. I would preside as a Friendly Fellow, speaking in non-plummy tones and sounding, hopefully, like an unaffected, intelligent, personable human being to whom new listeners could conceivably relate.

We would neither dumb down nor smug up.

As a presenter, I would neither berate nor patronise. I would be human. This was new.

This was the plan. I was happy and confident that we were breaking new ground by rendering Radio 4 accessible to a wider range of people, acknowledging that there was life beyond the chattering classes. We were out to win the culturally disenfranchised.

The birth of the new series was trumpeted by the rolling Radio 4 publicity machine and I succumbed to polite interviews from representatives of worthy publications. The outlook was positive.

Everything went according to plan, and on the day of our

first broadcast I awoke with a light heart and a tingle of anticipation. It was Monday 21 February 1994.

Those around me were nervous. I, on the other hand, was an oasis of calm. I was used to this pressure from live television, where one learns to distance oneself from the confusion and panic that is the norm on any show of this nature.

I adopted my usual state of suspended animation.

With anxious eyes staring wildly at me through the glass of the studio control-room, I calmly waited for our carefully selected signature tune to ebb, opened my mouth and spoke in what I hoped was a calm, reassuring and confident manner.

We had assembled a variety of items. To emphasise our brief, we had gathered some young people in an antechamber outside the studio, where an attractive linguist called Alison would expose them to an hour's crash course on regional accents, particularly the Geordie variety. Over the course of the hour-long programme, I would flit to and fro checking on progress made, asking questions about diphthongs and glottal stops.

Educate, inform and entertain. The Reithian way.

We had experts in the studio to examine the theory that fathers living at home were not necessary for the proper rearing of children. This would encourage phone calls. Irate or otherwise.

We had a fifteen-minute recorded piece charting a day in the life of two private investigators who were staking out an insurance fraudster. I thought this was particularly well done and felt the need to congratulate those who had recorded it. It was award-winning work.

We also had a feature on the changing smell of Grimsby, once a top-of-the-range, reeking fishing port but which was now blessed with other alien odours. Try finding that on another radio station.

Hundreds of listeners phoned the programme to take part in our parenthood discussion, and we put as many of them on air as possible. As I had hoped, the calls came from all over the country. I revelled in the variety of accents. Hands across the country. My adrenalin level rose and I was cookin'.

All went smoothly. At the end of the programme, I was pleased. It was *Woman's Hour* for both sexes. Not a bad thing. I was confident that we had pulled it off. We were on the right track. We were rolling.

Those involved were on a high, and evacuated the studios to swig celebratory first-show drinks in upstairs offices. We were joined by members of the BBC hierarchy, who congratulated us heartily, although I did notice that one of the suits was eyeing me in a peculiar manner.

The programme continued happily for a couple of weeks. I continued to take many phone calls on air, talking about racial stereotypes, spoilt children, time capsules, inner-city problems, the perils of bungee jumping and other topics that we knew would elicit comment from the listeners. We also continued to commission quality features, gave new writers and poets an opportunity to shine, and generally felt that we had something for everybody.

It felt good.

It was nice not having to worry about saying something that might get me killed.

It was nice talking normally to people without the need to employ even the slightest trace of showbiz bullshit.

It was nice to stretch out and relax in front of a nationwide, receptive audience.

It was nice to feel liked.

Except that I wasn't.

After three weeks there were rumblings from the Shires. Apparently the shock-waves had started almost immediately but had taken three weeks to gather serious momentum.

This came as a complete surprise to me, as we had had no flak from the people who rang the programme.

My first indication that there was something amiss came when I began to receive brochures from funeral parlours. I got one most days, the first from an undertaker in Eastbourne who wrote me a 'personalised' letter in reply to my alleged request for his services. It was a sombre brochure, colour photographs of reasonably priced coffins.

Amused, I browsed over the range and decided that, if pushed, I would be inclined to settle for the all-white teak model which seemed to have convenient air-holes, like the cardboard boxes that are used for transporting day-old chicks.

As my collection of brochures from country-wide undertakers multiplied, I realised that somebody was trying to tell me something.

This was new. I thought I'd had everything thrown at me in Northern Ireland, but this was a first. This was radio criticism at its most macabre. I counted fifty coffin catalogues before I lost interest and threw the new ones into the bin. I never did find out who had initiated them, nor did I want to. Irate callers rang the BBC and wrote many angry letters to *Feedback* (a Radio 4 letterbag programme) complaining about a decline in standards.

The programme was deemed a disgrace to Radio 4. How dare these common people phone a Radio 4 programme, and who was this slurring foreigner who let them speak on air? Why, sometimes he didn't even pronounce the 'g' at the end of his -ing words!

Well, pardon fuckin' me, I thought.

The heat intensified.

Sniffing the air, the 'quality' broadsheets joined the chase. First to strike were the radio critics, concerned about my 'provenance'.

I then graduated on to the editorial columns. They were calling shrilly for my head.

But why? I couldn't figure it out. What was it about a radio programme that could relegate vital affairs of state and vicious foreign wars to the back burner? Why were people so angry? Why was what I did so wounding to them?

I slowly realised that I had unwittingly scratched the

surface of something preternatural. I had roused a beast. The beast had assumed that I was questioning its values and was responding with vigorous swipes of its spiked tail.

I was witnessing the mobilisation of the Radio 4 Nazis. *Anderson Country's* mission was to make the network more accessible to others. The Nazis weren't having it.

I was in a state of some confusion, thinking I had missed something that was obvious to others. I listened as objectively as I could to the programmes we had done so far and found them perfectly acceptable. I was no fool. I knew what was good broadcasting and what wasn't. There was nothing there to justify the viciousness of the criticism.

I felt this was an unjust war.

Cries of rage continued to trumpet from retired civil servants in Brighton, old India hands harrumphed, and pink-haired ladies squealed that I should be sent back to Ireland where I belonged. They hated me passionately.

I wondered why. I didn't exactly expect to be loved, but why should I expect to be hated so intensely?

They said I was flippant and not serious enough.

I pleaded guilty on all counts. It's called being Irish.

Also, it became increasingly clear to me that many hardcore listeners seemed to feel that new listeners shouldn't be allowed to tune in to Radio 4 unless they sat a stiff examination.

However, what rattled me most was the considerable number of regular listeners who obviously thought that they were better than anybody else.

This kind of thinking was new to me.

Reporters were sent to look at me and scribble.

I remember one in particular. She was from a woman's magazine. I knew I was in trouble as soon as I saw her. Young, lank-haired, pimply-faced and flinty-eyed, she was Oxbridge and knew it, riddled with Penguin scholarship. A victim of a wasted education wearing comfortable shoes.

I tried to be nice to her but it was no good. She was

impervious to any overtures of civility. We settled in downy sofas. She glared long and hard, making me feel as if she had just witnessed me raping a pensioner.

Fuck it, I thought. I was probably in line for a shafting, so why be nice?

'What do you have to say to listeners who say that you shouldn't be on Radio 4?' she chirped.

'Well, I say this. If they don't like me they should flip the dial and listen to somebody else.'

She bristled. 'That's hardly the attitude.'

'Well, it happens to be mine.'

'Is that all you have to say?'

I cast away my Mae West. 'Yes, except to add that people like yourself should lighten up, open your minds a little and let other people breathe. And if that's too difficult, I could suggest remedial measures. The people who are shouting loudest should try a fortnight in Majorca. Get themselves a jug of sangria and a Big Mac. Do them the world of good. Might chill them out.'

Her eyes blazed with anger and her mouth shaped what I guessed to be the beginning of the phrase 'How dare you!' She thought better of it, bit her lip and dug a pencil deeply into her stylish notebook.

The interview ended. She left without saying goodbye and skewered me in her article. Amongst other things, she referred to me as 'The Most Hated Man In Britain'.

Gee, thanks.

I wondered if the Yorkshire Ripper had read the article. Probably would have cheered him up considerably.

I was past caring.

Meanwhile, panic broke out in the ranks. I took to sheltering in my office cutting bad reviews out of the newspapers, making little paper planes out of them and attempting to fly them into the waste-paper bin in the corner.

There seemed little else I could do.

I couldn't figure it out. I knew I was as good a broadcaster as anybody else (after all, people don't get Sony Gold Awards for whistling along with old Abba records). What annoyed me most was that the things I knew I was good at were the things that annoyed people most. I had no more arrows in my quiver.

There was a curious silence on the seventh floor.

'We're going to cut back on the phone calls,' I was told.

'And what'll we do instead?' I asked.

'More standard Radio 4 fare.'

'But I can't do that. That's like asking Alistair Cooke to host *Blankety-Blank*. Who do you want me to become? Jonathan Dimbleby? I'm genetically unsuited.'

'The programme's not working. You don't need me to tell you that.'

'Maybe it will in time. Maybe they'll get used to me.'

'The heat's too hot.'

'They'll crucify me if I pretend to be something that I'm not.'

'They're crucifying you now.'

'If I change, they'll smell blood and zone in for the kill.'

'They're doing that now.'

'Let's ride the bastard out. Let's keep doing what we're doing.'

'They'll picket the building. Your life won't be worth living. They'll hunt you like an animal.'

'So what do you suggest?'

'Sound more informed.'

'I am fucking informed.'

'Try to sound less populist. Sound more like a real Radio 4 presenter. We'll do more Radio 4-type material.'

I reluctantly agreed, beaten into submission by the unacceptable logic of it all. I had no fight left in me.

I suppose I should have resigned immediately. But I couldn't let this thing beat me. Stubborn.

I tried hard.

Thus followed nightmare months of talking to Sir Richard Rogers about the changing architecture of London, interminable discussions with Oxford dons on the 'essence of criticism', a filleting of the Cod Wars and a dissection of new theories on town planning. I was practically suicidal.

This was far from the programme we had envisaged.

Granted, the public furore died down somewhat, but not much. The radio critics on the broadsheets were not to be appeased, and continued to hammer away at every opportunity.

I was miserable. Confidence totally shot. It got to the point where I was afraid to open my mouth on air in case I mispronounced a word, knowing that such a slip would release the Hounds of Hell.

I was in the belly of the beast.

Each afternoon, stepping into the lift that would take me down to Studio B16 where the programme aired, I felt as if I were boarding the tumbril for Tyburn.

Everything I did was wrong.

The year before, I had written and broadcast a short series of monologues on Radio 4. These fifteen-minute talks had been received favourably, and one critic even went so far as to suggest that I could be the next Alistair Cooke (no thanks). This was interpreted as praise. Before *Anderson Country* started, I had recorded a second series, and although it is not my place to say that it was better than the first, it was certainly no worse.

Two months into *Anderson Country*, the second series was broadcast. The critics who had praised the first series un-animously declared the new programmes a load of crap.

The goalposts had been moved.

I considered taking to drink, but discarded it as an unviable option.

I offered to leave the programme but was urged to stay, on the grounds that the criticism would bottom out. After all, it couldn't possibly get much worse.

Months of torment followed. I began to feel physically sick at the prospect of broadcasting the programme, and experienced nausea and severe dizzy spells at increasingly frequent intervals.

I was convinced the programme was going to kill me.

I went to a doctor, who told me that he wasn't sure what was wrong with me. He sent me to a specialist, who told me that I possibly had Ménière's disease, urged me not to worry about it, gave me pills to encourage dehydration, and put me on a salt-free diet in a bid to stop me falling over.

This is all I fucking need, I thought. My career's going down the toilet and now I have a disease that'll drain my body of essential fluids and make me fall down in the street.

However, I was determined not to miss a programme.

Don't give in to the bastards.

I travelled home to Northern Ireland every weekend. My old colleagues looked at me as if I were a diseased dog that should be put down. They were, however, sympathetic, and made encouraging noises.

I was distraught.

I still had my Friday-night television talk-shows. I had hitherto regarded this task as somewhat stressful, but compared with what was going on in England, live television was positively relaxing. Nevertheless, my new-found lack of confidence easily transferred to the small screen.

One Saturday night at home in Stroke City I was unwinding in a local bar. Having taken a drop too much, I tottered towards the gents and bumped into a fellow BBC employee.

'What's going on over there?' he asked cheerily. 'Are they going to get you or what?'

'You should be rooting for me,' I replied thickly. 'I'm paving the way for bastards like you. I'm a pioneer.'

'You know what happens to pioneers?' he replied.

'Wha?'

'Indians scalp them.'

Well, yes.

The year dragged interminably by. I was determined to make *Anderson Country* work without selling my soul. Once or twice I pronounced the 'g' at the end of my -ing words. But I felt that even this was too much of a compromise. I was determined to be accepted on my own terms. In weak moments, I tried to be less flippant and, in desperation, once experimented with a new braying laugh that I knew was popular on Radio 4. Shamed by this, I decided to try no more. If they didn't like me the way I was, I wasn't going to try to be somebody else.

Although I must admit that, towards the end of my stint, I couldn't have sounded more informed if I'd swallowed the entire contents of the new British Library.

It made no difference.

The Home Counties Nazis wanted me out.

Came the inevitable. The BBC suits were eventually worn down by the volley of abuse from Middle England and it was gently explained to me that the burden of presenting a show like this was 'too much for any one man'. And who could blame them? The Blitzkrieg was unweatherable.

So. *C'est la guerre.*

After nearly a year of hell.

Hounded out of England.

On my departure, a radio critic on one of the 'quality' Sunday newspapers headed his column, 'Gotcha, Gerry!'

It all became clear.

I was the *Belgrano*.

THE ARGENTINIAN
RETURNS

I HAVE BEEN back home for some time.

It is late 1998. An uneasy peace holds sway in Northern Ireland.

I am taking the air on a cold, blustery afternoon.

A barefooted, half-naked man with a bullet-shaped head sways unsteadily near the entrance to a dilapidated church. He counts the coins that are clutched in his grimy hand.

As I walk past, he stumbles towards me. In any other city I would expect him to ask me for money. But no, this is Stroke City.

He asks me for a French kiss.

I show no sign of alarm and politely refuse. It's the only way. I suggest that fifty pence would be more beneficial to him. He reluctantly agrees. As I grease his palm with the silver, he informs me that Jesus loves me.

I thank him and am allowed to proceed.

Just another day in Stroke City.

I see a ragged sign outside the disused church. It reads, 'Jesus Loves the Entire City'.

I recognise the need for assurance such as this, knowing as I do that otherwise sane and educated people believe that Jesus loves only those who live in certain areas of this troubled metropolis. These people are also convinced that Jesus regards the rest as scum.

Problem is, the scum believe that God is on *their* side.

This is a strange country. Nobody sees the Big Picture.

I once sat with a friend of mine and attempted to paint the Big Picture, metaphorically speaking, of course. Some years ago, he had taken part in an exercise of community goodwill known as the Peace Train. On a yearly basis, Northern Ireland pacifists from opposing political and religious backgrounds would board this locomotive and chug happily between Belfast and Dublin in a bid to demonstrate to our brothers in the Republic of Ireland that the Northern Irish weren't all animals and could co-exist in an enlightened manner.

Unfortunately, during the course of one of these civilised excursions, a difference of opinion emerged between my friend and a fellow passenger which resulted in the latter being struck about the head by my friend's clenched fist.

I tried to explain to him that his behaviour had possibly undermined the thinking behind the concept of the Peace Train and that a full-scale punch-up may not have been the desired outcome of the initiative. He remained unmoved and stood resolutely behind his belief that the other guy had deserved it.

There was no Big Picture.

Now that all is supposedly peaceful, our politicians say that they too have finally seen the Big Picture.

Former tub-thumpers and mob-handlers have bought shiny suits and all talk together under one roof.

This is progress.

This is democracy.

Let bygones be bygones.

Let's make a new start.

A fat representative of the people stands up and makes a speech on live television. Somewhere in the middle of it, he pauses and looks around at the assembled throng. A smile creases his porcine face, his jaw drops imperceptibly and a quizzical expression appears. The look that bank managers adopt when they are about to tell a joke.

His amusing aside takes the form of an announcement. He informs the room that the Northern Ireland Shooting Team have just won a gold medal in an international marksmanship competition. He knows this will be good for a laugh. Good old black humour, you see.

The TV cameras pan the politicians. All are laughing uproariously. Laughing loudest are those who are directly or indirectly responsible for the deaths, by shooting, of people who, had they lived, would now be their constituents. It's great fun. Thighs are slapped and sides are split.

The irony is surely not lost on the many television viewers at home, a fair proportion of whom have had sons, daughters, husbands, wives and other relatives killed as a direct result of the activities of some of these braying representatives. They watch, presumably stone-faced.

On other occasions, self-important local politicians urge the President of the United States to keep his nose out of Ulster's business.

Like horseflies whining about the swish of Arkle's tail.

But this is peacetime.

Let's do peacetime things.

I am on my way to a circus, a real circus.

I am to be Guest Ringmaster at a special charity performance.

I have never been a Guest Ringmaster before and am unsure of what is expected of me. The show is scheduled to start shortly. I mingle backstage with the performers whilst the real Ringmaster is summoned.

I find myself talking to a short Moroccan clown who is smoking an untipped cigarette and drinking Irish whiskey from a large glass. He offers me a sip. I accept.

He is wearing his full regalia: too-small bowler hat, revolving bow-tie, huge, hooped, striped trousers, Little Tich boots and in his lapel, a flower that squirts water. He offers me another drop of his whiskey. We swig and talk. A small monkey wearing similar clothing jumps on to his lap. We are not introduced.

The smoke from his cigarette swirls upwards into his prop red nose, causing him no apparent discomfort. Behind us we hear the revving of the clowns' small fire engine. Water is poured into buckets.

The clown tells me about his marital problems. He has two wives. He is not really a clown, he says. He's a trained acrobat. I know what he means.

He tells me that he likes Northern Ireland.

An Indian elephant takes a shite five yards away. The clown doesn't notice.

A shapely trapeze artist walks past. Her tights are frayed.

A miniature horse chomps on an apple. A llama strolls by.

The real Ringmaster appears and welcomes me. He looks and dresses like Liberace.

'What do you want me to do?' I ask.

'Don't worry. I'll do most of the show,' he says. 'Just introduce the occasional act. I'll give you the details.'

'What time am I on?' I ask.

He consults a piece of paper.

'You're on after the horses.'

Well, yes.

At the end of the show, all participants are invited back into the ring to receive applause.

An actress from *Coronation Street* is in town with a touring theatre company and has agreed to appear briefly at this benefit circus. Also present is a man from *The Bill* or some similar TV drama, I forget which.

The *Coronation Street* actress is greeted with hysteria, and stands beside me in the middle of the sawdust-covered ring, bowing repeatedly.

We are flanked by a performing seal and a shite-stained elephant.

The actress is trying to smile. Manages only a grimace.

I catch her eye and wink.

'Showbusiness, eh?' I say. 'Can you beat it?'

She does not reply.

*

After the circus I take a nostalgic walk through darkened Stroke City streets.

I come upon the city-centre area where I was born, near what was formerly known as 'Aggro Corner' on the fringe of the Bogside. All the old houses have gone. Involuntary demolition. Our old house was blown up accidentally by the IRA in 1971. My mother was in the house at the time. No time to get out.

The bomb went off. She emerged dust-covered but unhurt. It was one of those *Reader's Digest*-type miracle escapes. Life's like that.

She suffered no discernible harm except that she no longer appreciates surprises. Doesn't hear too well any more either. Bombs are loud.

The IRA contacted her later and apologised.

Sorry, missus.

She'd lived there for thirty years.

Tough.

I look down an alleyway near my home and remember a young man I knew who had died there.

He was in a pub one night with the wrong people.

He was a ladies' man. Bit of a dandy with a weakness for drink. He bragged about what he would do if he only had a chance. He declared himself ready to lay down his life for Ireland if the necessity arose.

It was the whiskey talking. That's all.

In a normal society this man would have been told to go home and sleep it off. Somebody might even have ordered him a taxi.

Not here.

Somebody gave him a loaded gun. He reeled out into the street waving the gun. Staggered down an alleyway towards a manned Army sangar.

Who can blame the young and probably terrified squaddie who aimed his rifle when he saw an armed man weaving his way firing at will?

The soldier did what soldiers are trained to do.

A drunk man lay dead in the alley.

I'm told that those who sent him to his death drank to his health.

Probably still do . . .